# Mnemonics
# and Study Tips
## for Medical Students

D0168645

# Mnemonics and Study Tips
## for Medical Students

# Two Zebras Borrowed My Car

## Second Edition

**Khalid Khan** BSc(Pharmacy) MRPharmS MBBS(London) MRCGP DRCOG DFFP DCH DCM(Beijing)

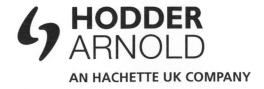

**HODDER**
ARNOLD

**AN HACHETTE UK COMPANY**

First published in Great Britain in 2003 by Arnold
This second edition published in 2008 by Hodder Arnold, an imprint of Hodder
Education, an Hachette UK Company, 338 Euston Road, London NW1 3BH

http://www.hoddereducation.com

Whilst the advice and information in this book are believed to be true and accurate at
the date of going to press, neither the author[s] nor the publisher can accept any legal
responsibility or liability for any errors or omissions that may be made. In particular,
(but without limiting the generality of the preceding disclaimer) every effort has been
made to check drug dosages; however it is still possible that errors have been missed.
Furthermore, dosage schedules are constantly being revised and new side-effects
recognized. For these reasons the reader is strongly urged to consult the drug
companies' printed instructions before administering any of the drugs recommended in
this book.

*British Library Cataloguing in Publication Data*
A catalogue record for this book is available from the British Library

*Library of Congress Cataloging-in-Publication Data*
A catalog record for this book is available from the Library of Congress

ISBN 978-0-340-95747-9

4 5 6 7 8 9 10

Commissioning Editor:       Sara Purdy
Project Editor:             Jane Tod
Production Controller:      Andre Sim
Cover Design:              Andrew Campling
Cover Illustration:        Bill Piggins
Indexer:                   Lisa Footitt

Typeset in Optima by Phoenix Photosetting, Chatham, Kent, UK
Printed and bound in India

What do you think about this book? Or any other Hodder Arnold title?
Please visit our website: www.hoddereducation.com

**mnemonic** /nemonik. L *mnemonicus* f. Gk *mnemonikos* derives from Mnemosyne, ancient Greek goddess. A memory aid or pertaining to aiding the memory. Often considered to be a code, device, acronym or formula to facilitate memory or understanding. The term is used here in its broadest possible sense.

Please return this book to:

# CONTENTS

*For the insatiably curious…*

## Q. So what exactly is a mnemonic?

The name comes from the Greek goddess of memory, Mnemosyne, the mother of the muses whose name means 'remembrance'. A mnemonic is essentially any type of memory aid – see above for a more precise definition. The term is used in the broadest possible sense, not only to include anagrams and codes, but also any tool or device that makes learning easier or more fun.

## Q. How is learning somebody else's mnemonic going to help me?

Given that they may have been used for generations, it's just possible that they will actually help. You'll remember your own mnemonics best because they'll be derived from the way your own mind works and will draw on your own particular strengths – hence some tips in Section III on making our own mnemonics. But you can still benefit from somebody else's knowledge or ideas – that's why you are at university in the first place!

## Q. Well, I know people who've never used a mnemonic in the whole of their medical career.

Then you haven't studied your paediatrics! The APGAR score is actually a mnemonic, and your first-aid treatment of sprains might be a bit rusty too (see RICE), not to mention a whole host of syndromes. Then there's ROY GBIV for the colours of the spectrum (or maybe the phrase Richard of York Gave Battle In Vain rings a bell?) and the well-known phrase Every Good Boy Deserves Football for musical sheets, etc. In fact medicine is replete with anagram-style mnemonics such as the many drug trials you know about. Another example is the modified Glasgow criteria for predicting severity of pancreatitis **PANCREAS** in which P stands for $PaO_2$ (< 8kPa); A for age (> 55); N for neutrophils $\neq$; C for calcium (< 2 mM); R for renal urea (> 16 mM); E for enzymes (LDH, lactate dehydrogenase > 6000 IU/L; AST, aspartate aminotransferase > 200 IU/L); A for albumin $\downarrow$; and S for sugar > 10 mM).

## Q. Why make revising medicine funny?

Humour is useful as a learning tool – just because something is serious doesn't mean it has to be miserable. Besides, humour coaxes your mind into producing more 'feel good' neurotransmitters, enhancing the learning experience – you are more likely to be interested in something you enjoy. In fact, humour has been used for centuries by doctors who are often exposed daily to the grimmest realities and horrors of human fragility. Humour is a coping mechanism and a release mechanism; it helps you keeps your sanity and allows you to give your best to your patients.

When a patient first sees you they have no idea of what you have seen or done just before their meeting with you – and neither should they – and they will still expect you to greet them warmly, hopefully with a smile, and ideally with a reassuring twinkle in your eye. If you feel good, so will they (just try looking totally miserable the next time you see a new patient and see how well that goes!). Peter Ustinov once said that comedy is simply a funny way of being serious.

**Q. So things like interest and humour help more than mnemonics?**

Exactly.

**Q. The effort of learning these acronyms in the first place makes mnemonics pointless. What on earth is SALFOPSM for instance?**

I agree. Not all of this type of mnemonic is easy or useful. I have attempted to limit the number of these to a few commonly used ones. They do become more useful if the first two letters are used, or if a rhyming word or phonetically similar letter is used – and you will notice plenty of these in this book. SALFOPSM is one mnemonic where you have to use a lot of effort to learn what it means and, although it is used by many students, I think it is quite difficult.

For the more curious among you, the branches of the external carotid artery are given by SALFOPSM thus: S for superior thyroid; A for posterior auricular; L for lingual; F for facial; O for occipital; P for posterior auricular; S for superior temporal; M for maxillary. And for the internal carotid you can use OPCAM – but I'll let you work that out for yourself.

**Q. I've read about short-term and long-term memory. Do memory aids have something to do with this?**

Yes. Generally most information enters your 'short-term' memory first and, then, by an unknown physiological process is stored permanently as a 'long-term' memory. All memory aids and systems work by linking your new information to an already existing piece of memory – something that you already know. In this process of association, the new knowledge gets a 'piggy-back' on the long-term memory, meaning you can assimilate the required knowledge quicker because your neurons have to make fewer new physiological changes (otherwise your brain would be making neuronal connections in a long-winded, tedious and random way).

**Q. So association is the basis of an efficient memory?**

Essentially, yes.

**Q. And you say that physiological changes actually happen when memories are made?**

Yes. The evidence for this has been accumulating for quite some time. One example is illustrated by the brains of London taxi-drivers. Researchers at University College London scanned the brains of sixteen cabbies and found that the hippocampus area (important anatomically in memory) became enlarged after they underwent 'knowledge' training.

**Q. What about dual-hemisphere brain-learning techniques?**

Well, the best way to learn is to use both hemispheres of the brain. This bilateral learning is coaxed and encouraged by the use of memory aids. It is inherent in the very nature of mnemonics. A good mnemonic will make use of the analytical and critical areas of your brain as well as the visual and creative parts – whether you like it or not. You will notice already that the more *modalities* you use (like smell, touch, and sight) the easier it is to remember things. The more extreme the sensory input, the more likely you are to remember it – the more vivid the picture, the stronger the smell, the more energetic the associated emotions, the stronger the connotations, the more powerful the memory will be, and the more likely it is to be 'written' directly in to your long-term physiological memory.

**Q. I find that the mnemonics disappear after a while, because I don't need them anymore... because I just know.**

Exactly! This happens when the facts become part of your long-term memory – you need mnemonic it no more – because you know more!

**Q. All the mnemonics I have heard are rude.**

They don't have to be rude or offensive to be useful – although sometimes this helps the associative process. Too many similar phrases defeat the object of the exercise, so I have not used many here. Although the rude ones can be very popular, they have their limitations as learning tools. Believe it or not, nowadays some students complain that they are not offensive enough!

**Q. But don't they just offend half the students while making the other half giggle?**

Actually the rudest, most offensive and explicit mnemonics I know about were supplied almost entirely by female medical students. Most of these are unpublishable, so I haven't included them here. Anyway, some don't make particularly good memory aids, especially because it can be confusing trying to remember who does what to whom!

**Q. I can't find this book in the medical school bookshop.**

Good grief! And this is THE most important text there is! Quick! Find the publisher's details!

**Q. What about mistakes?**

I quote Aeschylus (the ancient Greek playwright) who said: 'The wisest of the wise may err'. So apologies in advance – just in case. Anyway, these mnemonics do not replace your regular course notes, and they do not replace any existing or past guidelines or accepted clinical practices. They are simply to help with your revision. They do not replace clinical judgement or methodology, nor are they a substitute for any part of your training. But please do send your comments and/or point out any of the 'deliberate' mistakes! You can email email me at kk2@doctors.org.uk.

**Q. Why should I be making notes in the margin of this book?**

It will help you to learn. I have even left some space for your own scribbles. Jotting and doodling involve more areas of your brain, reinforcing the memories and crystallizing those thoughts in your mind. The process of using your hands in addition to both brain hemispheres contributes to whole-brain learning – and it will make you a better learner.

**Q. Have you kept all the interesting quotes?**

Confucius said: 'Study the past if you would divine the future.' That's what these quotes aim to do. Of course, another way to study the past is to look at previous exam papers or to ask students in the year above you how they passed last year! As you know, interesting anecdotes help to keep you stimulated, so you are more motivated to keep learning.

**Q. So as I read and learn, this book – funny, yet serious – will show me techniques for association and how to use humour to evoke interest and stimulate my neurological memory to its fullest potential, while also giving me the tools to devise my own mnemonics and study techniques, so maximizing the efficiency of my revision time?**

Exactly! Well said!

**Q. And there are no rules in mnemonics, except to do what works?**

Precisely!

**KK 2008**

# WHY *THIS* BOOK IS SO GOOD!

Congratulations! You are a student of one of the most exciting undergraduate courses in the world. Time and knowledge are precious; you will be challenged in countless directions, with constant syllabus changes, and you will be expected to assimilate a colossal amount of raw knowledge. Therefore, you need to manage your time and energies efficiently. Herein lies some assistance.

This compilation of medical mnemonics places the emphasis on user-friendliness. Those that are quickest to assimilate are given priority, so many popular, old favourites are included, and there is guidance on how to study efficiently and create your own memory aids. You will remember many of these forever, and with minimal effort. Remember, this book will be there for you all the way from freshers to graduation and beyond...

Einstein said that if there is an easier way – find it! There are some easier ways in this magical volume. Go find 'em!

## Second Edition – *still* good!

Welcome to the second edition. The last one was the first British mnemonics book for nearly twenty years, introducing a raft of innovations such as contextualized cross-referenced mnemonics with their alternatives, special 'swot' boxes, limericks, study techniques, links, pegs and an shameless infusion of fun on every page. Even the colour of the ink was carefully chosen to be relaxing and meditative, to help keep you super-calm the night before an exam.

Recently there has been a surge of student-friendly books. Mnemonics are everywhere now and publishers are making far more 'enjoyable' products – long may this trend continue. Of course, mnemonics have been used for generations all over the world. For example, in China rhyming songs have been used to pass down memories for centuries. There are several effective new verses included here.

Well done to the publisher for taking the plunge at a time when no-one in the UK wanted to publish a book like this. Eighteen years after I introduced my early hand-written booklets at St Georges, the Students' Union is still producing the mnemonics book. In 1990, medical students thought 'mnemonic' was a chest condition! (That's why we always include a definition of the word at the beginning of the book.)

All the mnemonics in this book have been used or 'tested' in the field, on medical students from various schools, and they all 'work' – but you must pick and choose what works best for you. Even better – make your own.

Anything that makes learning quick and fun and magical is always welcome.

**KK 2008**

# ACKNOWLEDGEMENTS

This publication would not have been possible without the help, cooperation and encouragement of hundreds of students from various medical schools and colleges over many years. Although many of the innovators of mnemonics over the centuries will remain anonymous (and therefore cannot be specifically credited here), I wish in particular to give my thanks to following people:

Aamir Zafar
Aidan Mowbray
Amer Shoaib
Andrew Eldridge
Atique Imam
Caroline Hallett
Chris Menzies
Debbie Rogers
Dia Karanough
Dush Mital
Elizabeth Picton
Georgina Bentliffe
Hammad Malik
Harvey Chant
Helen Marsden
John Morlese
Kate Ward
Kevin Chua
Khalid Hassan
'Kuz'
Leigh Urwin

Mahmooda Qureshi
Majeed Musalam
Matt Jones
Megan Morris
Milan Radia
Nazneen Ala
Neil Bhatia
Paul Kennedy
Paul McCoubrie
Paul Roome
Quinn Scobies
Raj Bhargava
'Rats'
Raza Toosey
Rob Ward
Dr Robert Clarke ('The Barnet course')
Sana Haroon
Shahid Khan
Sheetle Shah
Sophie Shaw
Stuart McCorkel

Thanks also to the General Management Committee of the St George's Hospital Medical School Club. My special thanks go to Dr Aftab Ala.

Every effort has been made to trace the original sources and copyright holders and to cite them in this book, but in this large compilation we recognize this has not always been possible. Those we have not included citations for are either anonymous, or no-one has declared ownership of them! To this end, any individual who claims copyright for one of more

mnemonic in this book should contact the publisher, so that an acknowledgement may be included in future editions.

Please note that all characters in this book are entirely fictional and do not
in any way related to real persons, alive or dead. The only exceptions are
those people whose sayings or quotes I have given acknowledgement or
credit to.

# SECTION I

## BASIC MEDICAL SCIENCES

# Chapter One

# ANATOMY

*Anatomy is destiny*

Sigmund Freud

*Our adventure begins with anatomy – where most students of medicine first come across mnemonics. Try this short quiz before you start reading:*

## ? PRE-QUIZ

1 Can you name the carpal bones?
2 What is the nerve supply to the diaphragm?
3 What are the posterior relations of the kidney?
4 Which palmar interossei abduct?
5 Which structures pass through the lesser sciatic foramen?
6 Which pain fibres carry crude touch sensations?
7 Which modalities are carried in the dorsal columns?
8 How many dermatomes do you know?

# 1.1 THE UPPER LIMB

## Rotator cuff

To remember the rotator cuff, think of the word 'sits'. This describes how the attachments of the rotator cuff muscles to the humerus.

SItS[1]

S        **Supraspinatus**
I        **Infraspinatus**
t        **teres minor**
S        **Subscapularis**

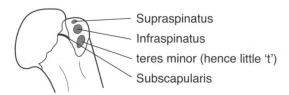

Supraspinatus
Infraspinatus
teres minor (hence little 't')
Subscapularis

# Latissimus dorsi

This is an old, anonymous and easy way of remembering that the latissimus dorsi muscle is attached to the humerus, on the floor of the bicipital groove, with the tendon between the attachments of the pectoralis major and teres major.

### Lady Doris Between Two Majors

**Lady Doris**    latissimus **d**orsi
(between)         (between)
Two **Majors**    pectoralis **major** and teres **major**

# Cubital fossa

Some students visualise Madeline Brown's Big Red Pustule to remember features of the cubital fossa. From medial to lateral, embedded in fat, you will find the median nerve, brachial artery, biceps tendon, radial nerve and posterior interosseous nerve.

### Madeline Brown's Big Red Pustule

**Madeline**    **Median nerve**
**Brown's**     **Brachial artery**
**Big**         **Biceps tendon**
**Red**         **Radial nerve**
**Pustule**     **Posterior interosseous nerve**

1  An original from Atique Imam FRCS, 1987.

## *Alternatives*

Mr Brown Bites Rabbits Posteriorly
Madeline Brown's Big Radiology Posting
Madeline Brown's Big Red Pussy.

Note that these characters are purely fictitious and are not based on anybody who ever existed. Mr Brown's rabbit gave the author verbal permission.

# Interossei muscles of the hand

There are four palmar and four dorsal interossei. They all have ulnar nerve innervation. Think of PAD and DAB to help you remember what they do.[2]

### PAD and DAB

| | |
|---|---|
| **PAD** | **P**almar interossei **AD**duct |
| **DAB** | **D**orsal interossei **AB**duct |

# Carpal bones

The eight small bones in the wrist are arranged in two rows of four. Imagine the proximal row of the wrist (Latin = *carpus*), from lateral to medial. You will see the scaphoid, lunate, triquetral and pisiform. Then visualise the distal row, going the other way from medial to lateral: you will see the hamate, capitate, trapezoid, trapezium. Here is an old favourite for remembering their sequence.

### Sue Likes Terry's Pens – Her Cap's Too Tight

| | | |
|---|---|---|
| **Sue** | **Scaphoid** | |
| **Likes** | **Lunate** | |
| **Terry's** | **Triquetral** | **PROXIMAL ROW** |
| **Pens** | **Pisiform** | |
| | | |
| **Her** | **Hamate** | |
| **Cap's** | **Capitate** | |
| **Too** | **Trapezoid** | **DISTAL ROW** |
| **Tight** | **Trapezium** | |

2 From Keith L. Moore (1985) *Clinical Orientated Anatomy*, 2nd edn. Philadelphia: Williams and Wilkins.

Variations include changing the people's names or using alternatives to 'pen' and 'cap', but they are all too rude to print here! If this is still too difficult for you to remember, try this elegant version in which both rows of carpal bones go from lateral to medial.

## Some Lovers Try Positions That They Cannot Handle

| | | |
|---|---|---|
| Some | Scaphoid | |
| Lovers | Lunate | |
| Try | Triquetral | PROXIMAL ROW |
| Positions | Pisiform | |

| | | |
|---|---|---|
| That | Trapezium | |
| They | Trapezoid | |
| Cannot | Capitate | DISTAL ROW |
| Handle | Hamate | |

Locate on your own wrist to see which bone you can most easily remember. This action will help to reinforce the memory associations in your brain.

### SWOT BOX

Now is a good time to remind you that the scaphoid (in the snuffbox) is the most commonly shattered bone in the wrist (and sometimes is not seen on X-ray for some 2 weeks or so).

# 1.2 THE THORAX

## Diaphragm

This simple rhyming verse will always remind you that the nerve supply to the diaphragm is via the third, fourth and fifth cervical nerve roots.

**C 3, 4 and 5**
**Keep the diaphragm alive!**

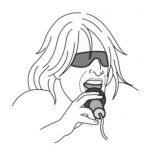

## Costal groove

The well-known sequence of important structures in the costal groove at the inferior border of the rib, going inferiorly, are the vein, artery and nerve.

**VAN**

| | |
|---|---|
| **V** | **Vein** |
| **A** | **Artery** |
| **N** | **Nerve** |

This is how these structures lie alongside a rib.

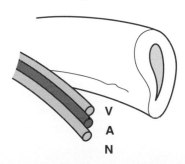

# Phrenic nerve

Here is the simple use of a pattern to make an association.

**The phrenic nerve**
**is in phront of the trachea**

# Lingual nerve

**The lingual nerve did a swerve**
**around the hyoglossus**
**Said Wharton's duct 'Well I'll be f****d**
**The bugger's double-crossed us!'**

(Several doctors and students contributed this one over the years so presumably it has been used a lot. Even though it has been around for decades, the original source has not been found.)

# 1.3 THE ABDOMEN AND PELVIS

## The kidney

The posterior relations of the kidney are similar on both sides of the body (the anterior relations are different).

 **SWOT BOX**

There is one artery – the subcostal. Two bones – the eleventh and twelfth ribs – are deep to the diaphragm. Three nerves – the subcostal, iliohypogastric and ilioinguinal – descend diagonally. Posteriorly, the superior pole of the kidney is related to four muscles – the diaphragm, the quadratus lumborum (more inferiorly), the psoas major (medially) and the transversus abdominis (laterally).

Try to remember this number sequence '1, 2, 3, 4' and this phrase 'all boys need muscle'. Now consider the following:

### 1-2-3-4 All Boys Need Muscle

1 **All**      **Artery**
2 **Boys**     **Bones**
3 **Need**     **Nerves**
4 **Muscle**   **Muscle**

## *Alternative*

A cheeky alternative for readers who are a lost cause is:

**Altered Boys Never Masturbate (and derivatives thereof).**

# Superior mesenteric artery

The superior mesenteric artery is one of those structures that arises at the level of the transpyloric plane and L1. It ends by anastamosing with one of its own branches – the ileocolic.

## MRI[3]

| | |
|---|---|
| **M** | **Mid-colic artery** |
| **R** | **Right colic artery** |
| **I** | **Ileocolic artery** |

# Renal arteries

To remember the branches of the renal arteries, cross your hands in front of you, at the wrist, as shown in the picture. The thumb represents the single posterior segment branch of the renal artery and the four fingers represent the four main anterior segmental arteries.[4]

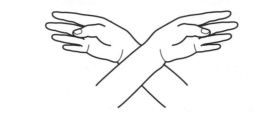

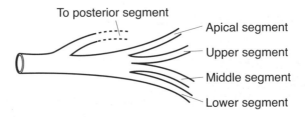

| | |
|---|---|
| **Thumb** | **Posterior segment branch** |
| **2nd Finger** | **Apical segment branch** |
| **3rd Finger** | **Upper segment branch** |
| **4th Finger** | **Middle segment branch** |
| **5th Finger** | **Lower segment branch** |

3  Attributed to Faisal Raza at University of East Anglia Medical School.
4  From John Blandy (1988) *Lecture Notes in Urology,* 4th edn. Oxford: Blackwell.

# The spleen

A useful description of the spleen (albeit in imperial measures!) is that it is 1 by 3 by 5 inches in size, it weighs 7 ounces and it lies obliquely between the ninth and eleventh ribs. To be able to regurgitate all this information, seamlessly, simply remember the number sequence.

**1-3-5-7-9-11**

| | |
|---|---|
| **1** | 1 inch |
| **3** | 3 inches |
| **5** | 5 inches |
| **7** | 7 ounces |
| **9** | 9th rib |
| **11** | 11th rib |

# Anal and urethral sphincters

You can remember that the second, third and fourth sacral nerve roots supply these sphincters from this simple rhyme.

**S 2, 3 and 4**
**Keep the pee off the floor!**

---

**!  NAUGHTY BIT**

Some authorities use a suitably 'shitty' word to describe the function of the anal sphincter. Choose whatever term you find most...*err*...convenient.

---

# 1.4 THE LOWER LIMB

## The thigh

There are five **adductor muscles** of the thigh – the pectineus, gracilis, adductor longus, adductor brevis and adductor magnus. These muscles are all supplied by the obturator nerve, except for the pectineus (femoral nerve). Part of the adductor magnus is also supplied by the sciatic nerve. They generally originate from the pubis. As well as adducting, they are important in fixating the hip joint and for normal gait. You will remember them with the help of this phrase.

### Observe Three Ducks Pecking Grass

| | |
|---|---|
| **Observe** | **Obturator** |
| **Three Ducks** | three **Add**uctors |
| **Pecking** | **Pectineus** |
| **Grass** | **Gracilus** |

 **SWOT BOX**

The gracilis (and its nerves and vessels) may be used surgically to repair damaged muscle. It is a relatively weak muscle and its loss has a minimal effect on leg adduction. Incidentally, tears or strains of the adductor muscles are common in fast bowlers (cricket) while ossification of the adductor longus can occur in horse riders.

Now consider the **posterior compartments** of the thigh. In ancient times these muscles (the hamstrings) were slashed in order to bring down enemy horses, and even to prevent prisoners from running away[5]! On a lighter note, here comes Swotty Samantha – note, she is a purely fictitious character.

---

5 From Keith L. Moore (1985) *Clinical Orientated Anatomy*, 2nd edn. Philadelphia: Williams and Wilkins.

### Big Fat Swotty Samantha Ate My Hamster's Pens

| | |
|---|---|
| **Big fat** | **Biceps femoris** |
| **Swotty** | **Semitendinous** |
| **Samantha** | **Semimembranous** |
| **Ate my** | **Adductor magnus** |
| **Hamster's pens** | **Hamstring portion** |

# Lesser sciatic foramen

This mnemonic will remind you that the nerve to the obturator internus, and its tendon and pudendal nerve and pudendal vessels pass through the lesser sciatic foramen.

### No Internals Tonight, Padre

| | |
|---|---|
| **No Internals** | **Nerve to obturator Internus** |
| **Tonight** | **Tendon** |
| **Padre** | **Pudendal nerve/vessels** |

# Sartorius and gracilis muscles

This elegant memory aid has long been used to remind us that the sartorius and gracilis are attached to the medial surface of the tibia just before (i.e. anteriorly) to the semitendinosus.

### Say Grace Before Tea

| | |
|---|---|
| **Say** | **Sartorius** |
| **Grace** | **Gracilis** |
| **Before** | **Before** |
| **Tea** | **Semitendinosus** |

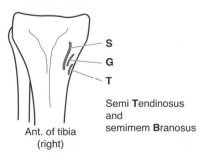

S
G
T

Semi **T**endinosus
and
semimem **B**ranosus

Ant. of tibia
(right)

# Supine or prone?

Any difficulty with these tricky terms is easily resolved with:

**Sup**ine – like a bowl of **soup**
**Pr**one – like doing **pr**ess-ups

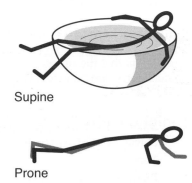

Supine

Prone

# The pelvis – Golly, is it male or female?

Just look at the shape of the greater sciatic notch to find out which is which.

**Lucy (female)**    **L-shaped sciatic notch**
**Johnnie (male)**    **J-shaped sciatic notch**

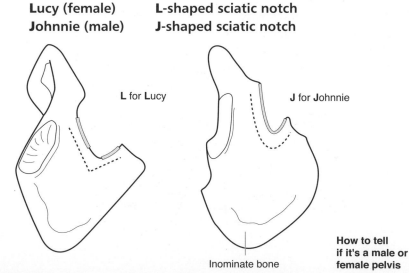

**L** for **L**ucy

**J** for **J**ohnnie

Inominate bone

**How to tell
if it's a male or
female pelvis**

# The patella – Is it a left one or a right one?

Place the patella with the posterior surface on the table in front of you with the inferior border (pointy corner) pointing away from you (distally). How it comes to rest on the table will show you whether it is from a left or a right knee.

Resting on its **right** side    From a **right** knee
Resting on its **left** side    From a **left** knee

# Ankle joint tendons

Inferior to the medial malleolus are the tendons of the tibialis posterior, flexor digitorum longus, posterior tibial artery, posterior tibial nerve and flexor hallucis longus.

### Tom, Dick and Harry

| | |
|---|---|
| Tom | Tibialis posterior |
| Dick | Flexor **d**igitorum longus |
| And | Posterior tibial **a**rtery and posterior tibial **n**erve |
| Harry | Flexor **h**allucis longus |

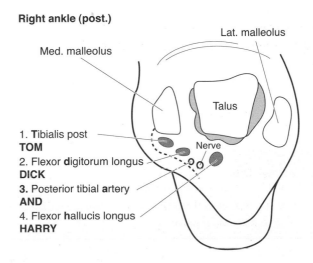

**Right ankle (post.)**

Lat. malleolus

Med. malleolus

Talus

1. **T**ibialis post
**TOM**

Nerve

2. Flexor **d**igitorum longus
**DICK**

**3.** Posterior tibial **a**rtery
**AND**

4. Flexor **h**allucis longus
**HARRY**

# The femoral triangle

The femoral triangle can be found as a depression inferior to the inguinal ligament (the base of the femoral triangle). Medially is the adductor longus and laterally is the sartorius (this is more obvious if the thigh is flexed, abducted and laterally rotated).

It is handy when you need to take blood via a femoral 'stab' or perform left cardiac angiographies to think of the word NAVY (but you do need to know where your Y-fronts are for this to work!).

## NAVY

| | |
|---|---|
| **N** | **Nerve** |
| **A** | **Artery** |
| **V** | **Vein** |
| **Y** | **Y-fronts** |

R

Nerve
Artery
Vein
Y- fronts !!!

And going medial to lateral, the floor of the triangle consists of the pectineus, iliacus, and psoas major – giving you PIMP.

## PIMP

| | |
|---|---|
| **P** | **Pectineus** |
| **I** | **Iliacus** |
| **MP** | **Psoas major** |

# 1.5 THE HEAD AND NECK

## Layers of the scalp

This is a very popular mnemonic judging by the number of texts it is quoted in – and justifiably so.

### SCALP

| | |
|---|---|
| S | Skin |
| C | Connective tissue |
| A | Aponeurosis |
| L | Loose connective tissue |
| P | Periosteum |

## Foramen magnum

The important structures passing through the foramen magnum are easily remembered by this phrase – as long as you say it with a German accent! Helpful in a clinch (but no apologies if it isn't!).

### Limp Sympathetic Men Vear Corduroy Accessories

| | |
|---|---|
| Limp | Meningeal **lymph**atics |
| Sympathetic | **Sympathetic** plexus (on the vertebral arteries) |
| Men | **Men**inges |
| Vear | **V**ertebral arteries (+spinal branches |
| Corduroy | Spinal **Cord** |
| Accessories | **Accessory** nerves |

## Foramens of Luschka and Magendie

The roof of the fourth ventricle has three foramens – the medial foramen of Magendie and two foramens of Luschka. The cerebrospinal fluid leaves via these openings into the subarachnoid space. This is how to remember the location of these foramens.[6]

| | |
|---|---|
| Magendie | Medial |
| Luschka | Lateral |

6 From Gertz SD, Gaithersburg MD (1996) *Liebman's Neuroanatomy Made Easy and Understandable*, 3rd edn. Aspen Publishers.

# Cranial fossa foramens

There are four middle cranial fossa openings, one of which is the **superior orbital fissure**.

The structures passing through the **superior orbital fissure** are the lacrimal nerve, frontal nerve, trochlear nerve, the superior division of cranial nerve III, oculomotor nerve (to superior oblique), nasociliary nerve, the inferior division of cranial nerve III and the abducens nerve (VI). A very old, oft-quoted mnemonic is:

### Lazy French Tarts Sprawl Naked In Anticipation

| | |
|---|---|
| **Lazy** | **Lacrimal** |
| **French** | **Frontal** |
| **Tarts** | **Trochlear** |
| **Sprawl** | **Superior division of III (nerve to superior oblique) – oculomotor** |
| **Naked** | **Nasociliary** |
| **In** | **Inferior division of III** |
| **Anticipation** | **Abducens** |

 **SWOT BOX**

The **superior orbital fissure** lies between the lateral wall and the roof of the orbit. It allows structures to communicate with the middle cranial fossa. A penetrating injury to the eye can therefore enter the middle cranial fossa and the frontal lobe of the brain. The superior orbital fissure meets the inferior orbital fissure at the apex of the orbit.

The other three main openings of the middle cranial fossa are the **foramen rotundum**, **ovale** and **spinosum**; the first two are in the greater wing of the sphenoid and the third (as its name suggests) is near the spine of the sphenoid.

### ROS

| | |
|---|---|
| **R** | Foramen **Rotundum** |
| **O** | Foramen **Ovale** |
| **S** | Foramen **Spinosum** |

# Maxillary nerve

There is also a neat way to remind yourself that the maxillary nerve exits the skull via the foramen rotundum and the mandibular nerve via the foramen ovale.

## Max Returns Mandy's Ovum…

| | |
|---|---|
| **MAX** | **MAX**illary nerve |
| **Returns** | foramen **R**otundum |
| **MANDy's** | **MAND**ibular nerve |
| **OVum** | foramen **OV**ale |

You can add another phrase to this to remind you that the important middle meningeal artery passes through the foramen spinosum, giving you 'Max Return's Mandy's Ovum…May Marry Spinster'.

## …May Marry Spinster

| | |
|---|---|
| **May MAR**ry | **M**iddle **M**eningeal **AR**tery |
| **SPIN**ster | foramen **SPIN**osum |

# Parasympathetic ganglia

The four parasympathetic ganglia are the ciliary, otic, pterygopalatine and sub-mandibular. Here is a simple mnemonic to remember them.

## COPS

| | |
|---|---|
| **C** | **C**iliary |
| **O** | **O**tic |
| **P** | **P**terygopalatine |
| **S** | **S**ubmandibular |

If this is far too boring (and you are not the politically correct type) then perhaps this modified but rather unflattering phrase of sound-likes and initial letters will be more memorable to you.

## Silly Old People stay Mouldy

| | |
|---|---|
| **Silly** | **C**iliary |
| **Old** | **O**ptic |
| **People** | **P**terygopalatine |
| **Stay Mouldy** | **S**ub**M**andibular |

**SWOT BOX**

The ciliary ganglion is in the posterior orbit. The oculomotor nerve (III) goes here too. Postganglionic fibres supply the ciliary muscle and pupils. The hypoglossal (IX) nerve supplies the otic ganglion and connects to the parotid gland, causing salivation. The pterygopalatine (or sphenopalatine) ganglion lies in its own fossa; nerve fibres come from the facial nerve (VII), supplying the lacrimal, nasal and palatine glands. The submandibular ganglion has fibres from the facial nerve (VII); it supplies the sublingual and (you guessed it!) the submandibular glands.

# Circle of Willis

Have you met Willis the spider? Students often find it helpful to visualize a spider like this one, with a face, eight legs…and a Willis.[7]

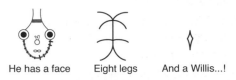

He has a face     Eight legs     And a Willis…!

And when you put them all together, it suddenly makes sense.

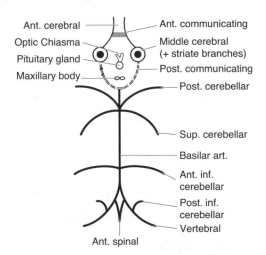

Don't forget that old exam favourite – the pontine branches.

7 Derived from a concept in Goldberg S (2007) *Clinical Anatomy Made Ridiculously Simple*. MedMaster.

**SWOT BOX**

The anterior cerebral arteries are involved in 30% of subarachnoid haemorrhages; the middle and posterior cerebral arteries each account for 25%.

# External carotid artery

I don't feel this anonymous mnemonic is especially good, however, it is undoubtedly favoured by some students.

### SALFOPSM

| | |
|---|---|
| S | **Superior thyroid** |
| A | **posterior Auricular** |
| L | **Lingual** |
| F | **Facial** |
| O | **Occipital** |
| P | **Posterior auricular** |
| S | **Superior temporal** |
| M | **Maxillary** |

How about creating your own (better) memory jogger for these structures.

# Carotid sheath

This is a portion of tubular cervical fascia enclosing the vagus nerve, carotid artery and internal jugular vein. AJAX is a quick way to remember what is in it.

### AJAX

| | |
|---|---|
| A | **Artery number 1 (the common carotid)** |
| J | **Jugular vein** |
| A | **Artery number 2 (the internal carotids)** |
| X | **Xth cranial nerve (the vagus)** |

NAVY works as a useful formula too.

## NAVY

| | |
|---|---|
| **N** | **Nerve (the vagus)** |
| **A** | **Arteries (the common and internal carotids)** |
| **V** | **Vein (the internal jugular)** |
| **Y** | **Y-shape (rough shape made by the two terminal branches of the common carotid artery)** |

 **SWOT BOX**

The carotid sheath extends from the base of the skull to the thorax. If the large vessels mentioned here are moved during surgery, the vagus nerve will be moved with them.

# 1.6 NEUROANATOMY AND NEUROSCIENCE

## Brain regions

A succinct reminder of the five major regions of the brain.

### Toddler's Messy Diapers Turn Yellow[8]

| | |
|---|---|
| **Toddlers** | **Telencephalon** |
| **Messy** | **Mesencephalon** |
| **Diapers** | **Diencephalon** |
| **Turn** | **meTencephalon** |
| **Yellow** | **mYencephalon** |

## Ventral and dorsal spinal columns

It is easy to remember that the grey ventral columns are motor.

| | |
|---|---|
| **Motor** | The **motor** is in the **front** (ventral) of most cars! |
| **Sensory** | Sensory modalities are dorSal |

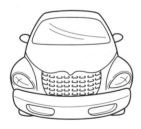

Also, to remind you of the sensory modalities (joint position, vibration, pressure, touch) which are in the dorsal (posterior) spinal column – take a look at Julie's Visible Panty Line.

### Julie's Visible Panty Line

| Julie's | Joint position |
| Visible | Vibration |
| Panty | Pressure |
| Line | Light touch |

# The cranial nerves

There are twelve cranial nerves, but how can you remember all their names, and with the right number? This helps, but again, use a German accent for best effect.[9]

### On Old Olympus's Towering Top, A Finn Vith German Viewed A House

| On | Olfactory | Ist cranial nerve |
| Old | Optic | IInd cranial nerve |
| Olympus's | Oculomotor | IIIrd cranial nerve |
| Towering | Trochlear | IVth cranial nerve |
| Top | Trigeminal | Vth cranial nerve |
| A | Abducens | VIth cranial nerve |
| Finn | Facial | VIIth cranial nerve |
| Vith | Vestibulocochlear | VIIIth cranial nerve |
| German | Glossopharyngeal | IXth cranial nerve |
| Viewed | Vagus | Xth cranial nerve |
| A | Accessory | XIth cranial nerve |
| House | Hypoglossal | XIIth cranial nerve |

How can one remember which ones are *sensory* or which are *motor* or which are *both*? Here's an easy way and well-known device:

9 Modified from Browse N, Black J, Burnand KG, Thomas WEG (2005) *Browse's Introduction to Symptoms and Signs of Surgical Disease*, 4th edn. London: Arnold.

## Some Say Marry Money But My Bride Says Big Balls Matter More

| Some | Sensory | Ist cranial nerve |
|------|---------|-------------------|
| Say | Sensory | IInd cranial nerve |
| Marry | Motor | IIIrd cranial nerve |
| Money | Motor | IVth cranial nerve |
| But | Both | Vth cranial nerve |
| My | Motor | VIth cranial nerve |
| Bride | Both | VIIth cranial nerve |
| Says | Sensory | VIIIth cranial nerve |
| Big | Both | IXth cranial nerve |
| Balls | Both | Xth cranial nerve |
| Matter | Motor | XIth cranial nerve |
| More | Motor | XIIth cranial nerve |

## *Alternatives*

On Occasion Our Trusty Truck Acts Funny (Very Good Vehicle, Any How). Attributed to Arvinder Singh of Ipoh, Perak, Malaysia. But most students seem to prefer this anonymous (rude) version: Oh, Oh, Oh, To Touch and Feel Virgin Girls' Vaginas and Hymens.

Take a look at a really effective way to learn this list using the 'peg system' as described in Section III.

# Extraocular muscle innervation

Consider the following 'formula' to describe the innervation of these eye muscles.[10]

## LR6 (SO4) 3

| LR6 | Lateral Recti | 6th (VIth) cranial nerve (abducens) |
|-----|---------------|-------------------------------------|
| SO4 | Superior Oblique | 4th (IVth) cranial nerve (trochlear) |
| 3 | All other extraocular eye muscles | 3rd (IIIrd) cranial nerve (oculomotor) |

10 Derived from Smith A (1972) *Irving's Anatomy Mnemonics.* Edinburgh: Churchill Livingston.

You now know the entire cranial innervation of the extraocular eye muscles – oh, you little genius! (And you can also remember that the *abducens* nerve *abducts* the eye.)

# Facial (VII) nerve

Branches are:

### Two Zebras Buggered My Cat

| | |
|---|---|
| **Two** | **Temporal** |
| **Zebras** | **Zygomatic** |
| **Buggered** | **Buccal** |
| **My** | **Mandibular** |
| **Cat** | **Cervical** |

## *Note*

No cats (or zebras!) were harmed in the making of this book!

## *Alternative*

The less risqué version is shown on the cover: Two Zebras Borrowed My Car.

 **SWOT BOX**

The facial nerve exits the skull via the stylomastoid foramen then runs superficially within the parotid gland before dividing into five terminal branches which supply the muscles of facial expression. The mastoid process is not present at birth, thus a difficult labour or use of forceps may injure the facial nerve.

The superior part of the motor nucleus of the facial nerve has bilateral cortical innervation, hence the muscles of the upper part of the face have a bilateral nerve supply – which means that in a an upper-motorneuron lesion there is contralateral paralysis of the lower half of the face (though the patient will still be able to close their eyes and wrinkle their forehead muscles). With a lower-motorneuron lesion (e.g. Bell's palsy) movement will be affected on the same side as the lesion.

**NAUGHTY BIT**

What do the chorda tympanae (facial nerve branch) and the clitoris have in common?

*(For the answer turn to next page – any physical action will reinforce the information you are learning!)*

# Vestibulocochlear (VIII) nerve – a test

A test for the vestibular division of the VIIIth nerve involves pouring cold or warm water into the external auditory meatus (ear hole) to bring about a temperature change. This temperature change affects the movement of endolymph in the semicircular ducts, and stimulates the hair cells (movement sensors) of the cristae. This in turn stimulates the vestibular nerve via the oculogyric nuclei in the brainstem, and causes nystagmus. Cold water causes nystagmus in the direction of the opposite eye; and warm water in the direction of the same eye. You can remember this with the COWS mnemonic.

## COWS

C–O        **Cold water – Opposite eye**

W–S        **Warm water – Same eye**

 **SWOT BOX**

Remember, the conventional direction of nystagmus is considered to be the direction of the 'quick' flick. In nystagmus, the eye wanders off, out of control. Your neurology attempts to correct it by flicking the eye back into position, so it can fixate on the on object being looked at.

> *Wear a smile and have friends*
> *Wear a frown and have wrinkles*
>
> George Eliot

# Pain fibres

Here is a useful way to remember the differences between A and C pain fibres.

| | |
|---|---|
| **'C' fibres** | **Carry Crude touch** |
| **'A' fibres** | **Pain Arises Abruptly and is blocked by Asphyxia** |

 **SWOT BOX**

C fibres are involved with pain that typically arises slowly and is poorly localized, often with a burning and unpleasant or disagreeable sensation.

A fibres are involved with pain that typically arises abruptly and is well localized, often with a sharp or prickling sensation. (Come to think of it, they have a lot in common with getting 'A' grades too.)

# Dermatomes – made easier

Imagine (to switch on the right side of your brain) a four-legged mammal, rather than a biped – this makes understanding the dermatomes much easier. Now, start at C1 and work your way down.

- C1 to C4 go to the head, neck and shoulders.
- C5 to T1 'disappear' as they 'wander off' to innervate the upper limb.
- T4 supplies the nipples.
- T10 supplies the umbilicus (see below).
- T12 is the lowest abdominal dermatome.
- L1 to S1 go to the lower limb.
- S2 to S5 are the only ones left for the bottom end.

If you study the following diagram and transpose it to a person standing upright, you will see the way the dermatomes flow. Go with that flow!

*ANSWER: They both supply taste to the anterior two-thirds of the tongue. (Awful, isn't it! And anonymous – not surprisingly!)*

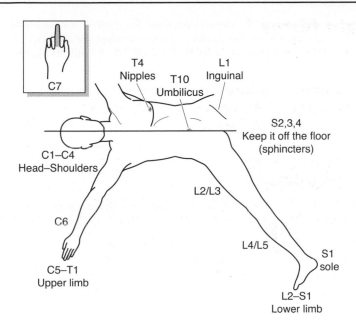

And more about the cervical dermatomes:

**One cervical, two cervical, three cervical, four, down the upper limb to find any more**

**Hold out your arms like a crucifix, stick up your thumbs – you have C6**

**Now wiggle C7 – the middle finger to heaven**

**And easy to extrapolate – ring and little fingers are C8!**

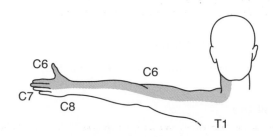

Some mnemonics for the dermatomes use the digit '1' instead of the letter 'I'. The dermatome to the axilla is T1 (remember the overlap of all the dermatomes). This is actually spelt out in the word 'armpit' like this:

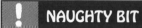

> ## ! NAUGHTY BIT
> Remember T4 = T **for** tits!

### T10 umbilicus

Did you know that the umbilicus is already *labelled* with its respective dermatome? Not convinced? Do I have to show you a diagram? OK here it is…*but for the rest of your life you will remember* that T10 innervates the umbilicus…

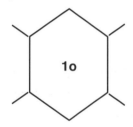

### T1 – armp1T

Dermatome L1 is spelt out in 'inguinal' as shown below. Thinking of this will also remind you that it is the **L**ast abdominal dermatome.

### L1 – 1nguinaL

For L3 remember this is roughly where cowboys holster their guns, and remember this rhyme too:

### L3 – goes to the medial knee

As for the first sacral nerve, S1, this supplies the little toes and the sole of the foot. Get it?!

### S1 – 1 Small toe

Or:

## S1 – So1e

Finally S2 to S4 relate to the sphincters, thus:

## S2,3,4 – keep it off the floor

You have now learned, with the minimum effort, most of the major dermatomes. Once you know a few of the key ones, you can extrapolate the rest. Remember that each dermatome *overlaps* with those above and below, which makes your revision even easier because you know the dermatome just above and below will be involved.

Another useful way of looking at the sacral dermatomes is summarized here:[11]

**You stand on S1**
**Lie on S2**
**Sit on S3**
**Wipe S4**
**Poke S5 (rectum)**

Review your knowledge of them with the song below, which ties all of this together. Remember that reviewing is a major key to success.

## The dermatome song

**One cervical, two cervical, three cervical, four, down the upper limb to find any more**

**Hold out your arms like a crucifix, stick up your thumbs – you have C6**

**Now wiggle C7 – the middle finger to heaven**

**And easy to extrapolate – ring and little fingers are C8!**

**T1 spelt in Armp1T is – as for nipples, well T(4) for tits**

**One dermatome ready labelled for us, T10 in the umbilicus!**

**L1 you know-it-all, 'cos it's spelt 1nguinaL**

**L3 to holster guns, you see, also goes to medial knee**

11 Contributed by Dr Laura Colvin.

L4 flows across the kneecap, but won't stop there, the busy chap,

It goes to make your bunion jingle – and with L5 the big toe tingle!

So to S1 and 1 small toe, a dermatome full of So1e

S2 on which you lie, S3 upon which you sit

S4 is what you wipe, S5 – put yer finger in it!

Perhaps not the most elegant of poems, but at least you know more dermatomes than you did five minutes ago!

# Chapter Two

# BIOCHEMISTRY

*These tips and suggestions will help with your
biochemistry revision. Try this first:*

---

**? PRE-QUIZ**

1  How many rings are there in the adenine nucleotide?
2  Which are the pyrimidine nucleotide bases?
3  How many hydrogen bonds are there between guanine and
   cytosine?
4  What are the four fates of pyruvate?
5  Can you draw the Lineweaver–Burke plot of competitive
   inhibition?
6  How many essential amino acids are there? Can you name
   them?

---

## Pyruvate metabolism

The four fates of pyruvate are given by GALA and are shown in the diagram
below.

**GALA**

| | |
|---|---|
| **G** | **Glucose** |
| **A** | **Alanine** |
| **L** | **Lactate** |
| **A** | **Acetyl coenzyme A** |

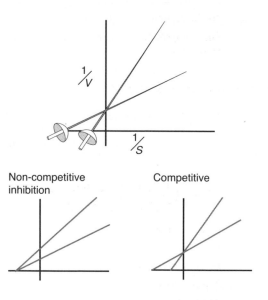

Glucose

aerobic

Acetyl-Co-A ◄——————► Pyruvate ——————► Alanine

anaerobic

ethanol in
some yeast

Lactate

# Enzyme inhibition

The Lineweaver–Burke plot is a graph showing competitive inhibition between two enzymes (below right). You can remember this by visualising two crossed swords – in competition. In non-competitive inhibition, they do not cross.

$\frac{1}{V}$

$\frac{1}{S}$

Non-competitive
inhibition

Competitive

# The cell cycle

The five phases of cell mitosis are encompassed by the IPMAT mnemonic.

## IPMAT

| I | Interphase |
| P | Prophase |
| M | Metaphase |
| A | Anaphase |
| T | Telophase |

The many stages of meiosis are remembered using PMAT–PMAT.

## PMAT–PMAT

| P | Prophase 1 |
| M | Metaphase 1 |
| A | Anaphase 1 |
| T | Telophase 1 |
| $P_2$ | Prophase 2 |
| $M_2$ | Metaphase 2 |
| $A_2$ | Anaphase 2 |
| $T_2$ | Telophase 2 |

# Essential amino acids

There are 20 amino acids in all but only 10 are *essential*. Eight of them are essential *always*, and two of them (histidine and arginine) are essential *only* in specific cases. The names of all 10 can be remembered by the following phrase.

### I Saw, He Phoned at 3:09 and Met Licentious Argentines – Lucy, Tracey and Val

| I saw | Isoleucine |
| He | Histidine |
| Phoned at | Phenylalanine |
| 3:09 | Threonine |
| Met | Methionine |
| Licentious | Lysine |
| Argentines | Arginine |
| Lucy | Leucine |
| Tracey and | Tryptophan |
| Val | Valine |

# Amino acid structure

The amino acids with *positive side chains* are given by HAL.

**HAL**

**H**  **Histidine**
**A**  **Arginine**
**L**  **Lysine**

Although the *R* group varies, you will probably know that *all* amino acids have this structure in common:

$$\underset{\displaystyle H_3N - C - COOH}{\overset{\displaystyle R}{|}}$$

Here are some handy aides for recalling the details about the structures of individual amino acids.

**Glycine**    **R = H (Hydrogen)**
            The simplest amino acid. We don't bother to write the letter **H** on chemical structures because the marked ends indicate hydrogen. So glycine's structure is the same as the above with the **R** bit left blank

**Alanine**    **R = CH$_3$ (Methyl group)**
            Hence 'It's all about **Me**, me, me…it's all-a-mine!' (*all-a-mine* rhymes with alanine)

**Valine**    **R = V-shaped group**
            The V-shape is shown in the diagram below. This makes it so easy – just stick a **V** up your **R**!

**Cystine**    **R = contains C–S (Sulphur attached to Carbon)**
            The clue is in the name **CyS**tine

**Leucine**     **R = looks like λ**
The Greek letter *lambda* (see below) gives us an 'L' sound for leucine

**Methionine**  **R = C–C–S–C**
What sounds will remind you of that? How about *cake-suck* or *Coxsackie's* (a virus)? How about a phrase like *methionine makes coke suck (-C-C-S-C)*

**Arginine**    **R = Pr–N–CNN (Propyl, Carbon, Nitrogen)**
Say *Argentina prayin' for CNN* to remind you of this side group

**Serine**      **R = CH$_2$OH (methanol)**
Think of a *searin'* pain caused by drinking methanol

**Threonine**   **R = EtOH (ethanol)**
Threonine has three oxygen atoms (*three-O*) and nine H atoms (*-nine*) – convenient, eh!

**Proline**     **R = ring-shaped Nitrogen-containing ring**
**R** is shaped like a **P**entago**N** with **N**itrogen in one corner – draw it out for yourself

# Lipids

Very-low-density lipoproteins (VLDLs) carry endogenous triglycerides from the liver to cells for storage for metabolism – these are the bad ones! High-density lipoproteins (HDLs) carry cholesterol away from the peripheral cells to liver for excretion – these are the good ones! Remember the difference like this:

| HDL | **H for Heroes** |
| VLDL | **V for Villains** |

# Redox reactions

This is an old school favourite – another anonymous one – about the loss of electrons in redox reactions.

**OIL RIG**

| | |
|---|---|
| **O** | **Oxidation** |
| **I** | **Is** |
| **L** | **Loss** |
| **R** | **Reduction** |
| **I** | **Is** |
| **G** | **Gain** |

# Stereoisomers

*Cis* molecules have both their R groups on the same side of a double bond, but *trans* molecules have them on opposite sides. Remember:

**Both on 'cis' side**

# Ortho, para and meta substitutions

*Ortho* means on position 2 of the aromatic ring. *Meta* means on position 3. *Para* is at position 4 and parallel to the carbon at position 1. To remember this easily, remember:

**Or-two met-a-tree para-four**

| | |
|---|---|
| **Or-two** | **Ortho-2** |
| **Meta a tree** | **Met-3** |
| **Para-four** | **Para-4** parallel to C1 |

# Huckle's rule of spatial stability

As you know, spatial stability is associated with six electrons. Well, it just so happens there are precisely the same number of letters in the word Huckle.

**6 electrons    6 letters in Huckle**

# Purine and pyrimidine nucleic acids

Nucleic acids are made up of a base, a five-carbon sugar and a phosphate group. The bases are either purines (two-ringed) adenine and guanine, or pyrimidines. The latter are the single-ringed thymine and cytosine (or uracil in RNA). Within the nucleic acid chain a pyrimidine always links with a purine and vice versa. So a DNA double-helix is *always* three rings wide.

### All Girls Are Pure and Wear Bras

| | |
|---|---|
| **All** | **Adenine** |
| **Girls are** | **Guanine** |
| **Pure** | **Purines** |

And to help you remember their structures:

**Purines are two-ringed structures...**
**...and so are bras!**

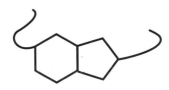

This leaves the single-ringed Pyrimidines, Thymine and Cytosine. You can try to visualize Pies, Tyres or Cytes (cells) to remind you of single-ring shapes, or perhaps a 'seat' for cytosine. Get the picture?

*Penser, c'est voir*
*(To think is to see)*

Louis Lambert

# Base-pairing

You will remember that the **nucleic acid** purine *only* pairs with a pyrimidine, giving a constant three-ring diameter to DNA. Use this rule:

### AT the GEC

| | |
|---|---|
| **AT the** | **Adenine only pairs with Thymine** |
| **GEC** | **Guanine links (via three hydrogen bonds) with Cytosine** |

This is ridiculously easy to remember if you think of the General Electric Company, the GEC, and if you know the E represents three hydrogen bonds:

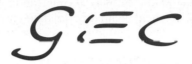

# The urea cycle

Several students claim that this anonymous mnemonic actually helped them learn the urea cycle (there is no accounting for taste!):

### Ordinarily Careless Crappers Are Also Frivolous About Urination

| | |
|---|---|
| **Ordinarily** | **Ornithine** |
| **Careless** | **Carbamoyl** |
| **Crappers** | **Citrulline** |
| **Are** | **Aspartate** |
| **Also** | **Arginosuccinate** |
| **Frivolous** | **Fumarate** |
| **About** | **Arginine** |
| **Urination** | **Urea** |

However, the biochemical cycles are probably best learnt by use of loci or peg mnemonics. See more on advanced mnemonics in Section III.

# Fat-soluble vitamins

### ADEK

| | |
|---|---|
| **A** | Vitamin **A** |
| **D** | Vitamin **D** |
| **E** | Vitamin **E** |
| **K** | Vitamin **K** |

# Chapter Three

# PHYSIOLOGY

*The first qualification for a physician is hopefulness*
James Little (1836–1885)

*How good is your knowledge of physiology right now?*

**? PRE-QUIZ**

1 Which are the five main excretory organs?
2 How many litres of interstitial fluid are there in an average adult?
3 Is ejaculation parasympathetic or sympathetic?
4 How is arterial blood pressure defined?
5 What effect does constriction of the iris have on the canal of Schlemm?
6 Is constriction of the iris sympathetic or parasympathetic?

## Blood pressure

'BP Copper' is a neat reminder of the relationship between **arterial blood pressure** (BP), cardiac output (CO) and peripheral resistance (PR).

### BP Copper
### $BP = CO \times PR$

If you ever get confused about whether **systolic pressure** or **diastolic pressure** is higher this think of 'S' for *squeezing* which is what the heart does during systole – hence giving a *higher* reading.

### Systolic pressure = Squeezing
### Diastolic = Dilating heart or D for down

# Anterior pituitary hormones

The **six anterior pituitary hormones** are thyroid-stimulating hormone (TSH), growth hormone (GH), the two gonadotrophins follicle-stimulating hormone (FSH) and luteinizing hormone (LH), prolactin (PRL) and adrenocorticotrophic hormone (ACTH).

## Those Giant Gonads Prolong the Action

| | |
|---|---|
| **THoSe** | **TSH** |
| **Giant** | **GH** |
| **Gonads** | **FSH/LH** |
| **PRoLong** the | **PRL** |
| **ACT**ion | **ACTH** |

# Immunoglobulins

There are five classes of Immunoglobulins – IgG, IgA, IgM, IgE and IgD.

## GAMED

**immunoglobulin G**
**immunoglobulin A**
**immunoglobulin M**
**immunoglobulin E**
**immunoglobulin D**

Each has four polypeptide chains – two heavy and two light. These chains are held together by disulphide (**S–S**) bonds. Heavy chains are specific to each class of Ig. IgM is produced first in the immune response. IgG appears later as the IgM level falls. This secondary response of IgG is due to activation of long-lived B lymphocytes on repeated exposure to the antigen. The secondary response is quicker and greater. Remember:

| | |
|---|---|
| **IgM** | **IM**mediately produced |
| **IgG** | **G**reater response |

# Ejaculation

Is ejaculation mediated by parasympathetic or sympathetic nerves? If you think of the erection as *pointing* and the ejaculation as shooting this makes perfect sense.[1] (Surely you don't need a diagram for this one.)

## Point and Shoot

| Point | Parasympathetic |
| Shoot | Sympathetic |

# Fluid compartments

This one needs a little bit of thought (stay calm – it's not too much). You need to say to yourself '1-2-3-30-45 if pit'. It works something like this:

## 1-2-3-30-45 ............... If Pit

| 12 litres | IF | Interstitial Fluid |
| 3 litres (plasma) | P | Plasma |
| 30 litres (inside cells) | I | Inside cells |
| 45 litres (total body water) | T | Total body water |

Do have a go. Contributed by an anonymous medical student, several others have found it helpful. Write it out a few times *now* and you will remember it. Writing will reinforce a motor memory and sensory pathway to strengthen the visual stimulus of the above.

# Excretory organs

Recalling the five main excretory organs is a SKILL well worth knowing!

## SKILL

| S | Skin |
| K | Kidneys |
| I | Intestines |
| L | Liver |
| L | Lungs |

1 With acknowledgement to P. McCoubrie and M. Jones, Saint George's Hospital Medical School, 1990.

# Canal of Schlemm

The canal is a space at the sclera–corneal junction. It drains the aqueous fluid away from the anterior chamber. Any increased resistance to this flow will cause a rise in intraocular pressure (IOP). Here's a handy way description:

## C.C.C.P.

| | |
|---|---|
| **C** | **Constriction of the** |
| **C** | **Circular muscle opens up the** |
| **C** | **Canal of Schlemm** |
| **P** | **Parasympathetically** |

 **SWOT BOX**

Friedrich S. Schlemm (1795–1858) was Professor of Anatomy in Berlin. He was **over 21** years old when he discovered the canal. By a freak coincidence, an IOP of **over 21** mmHg is a sign of glaucoma. Gotcha...! Now for the rest of your medical career you will know that an intraocular pressure **over 21** is a sign of glaucoma – whether or not you wanted to!

# Heart sounds

The first heart sound (S1) is made up of a mitral component (M1) and a tricuspid (T1) component (in order of valve closure). The second (S2) is made up of A2 (aortic) followed by the pulmonary valve closure (P2). This gives a sequence from S1 to S2 of M1–T1–A2–P2.

You will find this sequence easy to learn with 'Mighty Ape'.

## Mighty Ape

| | |
|---|---|
| **MighTy** | **M1 T1** |
| **APe** | **A2 P2** |

See page 83 for more on heart sounds and murmurs.

# Khalid's guide to the sarcomere

1. Draw two 'Z lines' – the borders of our 'Zarcomere'.

2. Draw an 'M line in the Middle.

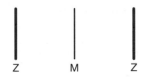

3. Add a dArk 'A' bAnd.

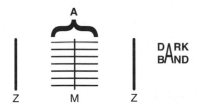

4. What's left must be the light 'I' zone.

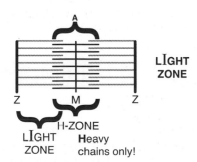

Simple!

# Chapter Four

# PHARMACOLOGY

*This chapter will be useful both in your physiology and pharmacology,
The section on receptors is relevant to your understanding
drug modes of action.*

## ? PRE-QUIZ

1 Are beta-1 receptors found predominantly in the lung or heart?
2 Can you name two non-adrenergic non-cholinergic
  neurotransmitters?
3 Which muscarinic receptors are more common in the brain?
4 What are the effects of beta-blockers on the lungs?
5 Is the above mediated by the sympathetic or parasympathetic
  system?
6 Is phenytoin used in the treatment of petit mal epilepsy?
7 Which prostaglandins dilate blood vessels?
8 What is the quadruple therapy of tuberculosis?

## 4.1 RECEPTOR REVISION

### Adrenoreceptors

In general, **alpha-stimulation** causes constriction of smooth muscles. A
handy way to remember this is to imagine the Greek letter $\alpha$ is made of
rope, so when the two ends are pulled it forms a tight knot.

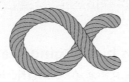

In general, **beta-stimulation** 'makes 'em bigger' meaning they cause the dilation of smooth muscles in structures such as the bronchioles, uterus, blood vessels. A good memory jogger is therefore:

### Beta makes 'em Bigger

And what about beta receptors in the **heart and lungs**? It's easy to learn which subtype predominates in each. The heart has predominantly beta-1 receptors, and the lungs have mainly beta-2, and of course you have one heart and two lungs. So:

### One Heart Two Lungs

| | |
|---|---|
| **One** heart | Beta **one** |
| **Two** lungs | Beta **two** |

Could it be any easier?

# Parasympathetic system

Here is a useful summary of the **gastrointestinal functions** of the parasympathetic nervous system:

### Periods Must Increase Secret Stomach Cramps

| | |
|---|---|
| **Periods** | **Parasympathetic system neuroeffector junctions are all...** |
| **Must** | **Muscarinic and...** |
| **Increase** | **Increase...** |
| **Secret** | **Secretions of the...** |
| **Stomach** | **Gastrointestinal system and...** |
| **Cramps** | **Gastric motility** |

Other systemic parasympathetic system effects are covered by this neat phrase:

### Decreased Arti's by Bringing Brad Pitt

| | |
|---|---|
| **Decreased** | **Reduction or constriction of...** |
| **Arti**'s by | **Art**erioles |
| **Br**inging | **Br**onchioles |
| **Brad** | **(Brad**y)cardia |
| **Pitt** | **P**upils |

## *Alternative*

**Bringing Brad's Pills Decreased Arti's.**

---

 **RAPID REVISION**

*Erection* is mediated **P**arasympathetically (**P**ointing) and ejaculation is mediated **S**ympathetically (**S**hooting) system. See p. 43.

---

From the central nervous system the first stop for all nerves are always *nicotinic* receptors. After that all **parasympathetic neuroeffector junctions** are *muscarinic* – thus the final stop is always muscarinic. Thus their path is spinal cord → nicotinic → muscarinic.

### Pat likes S'n'M

| | |
|---|---|
| **Pat likes** | **P**arasympathetic (nerves from the...) |
| **S** | **S**pinal cord (go via...) |
| **N** | **N**icotinic (then...) |
| **M** | **M**uscarinic |

# Muscarinic receptors

There are five subtypes ($M_1$ to $M_5$). As you now know, they are usually neuroeffectors for the parasympathetic system, peripherally, where they are found in smooth muscle and glands.

## MSG

| | |
|---|---|
| **M** | **Muscarinic (receptors peripherally are in...)** |
| **S** | **Smooth muscles (and...)** |
| **G** | **Glands** |

They are also very important centrally – especially the M₁ subtype. Generally they work by reducing cAMP (cyclic adenosine triphosphate). M₁ receptors are the most important and most widely expressed muscarinic receptors in the brain. M₂ receptors slow the heart down. M₃ receptors are the most important for bladder contraction.

This all ties together in the 'Muscarinic receptor song'.

### Muscarinic receptor song

| | |
|---|---|
| **Muscle-bound men are a little camp** | **Decreases cAMP** |
| My **big secret** makes you damp | **Increases secretions/** contraction |
| 'Coz... | |
| M3 makes me **pee**! | **Bladder** contraction |
| M2 **slows the heart**, dude | **Bradycardia** |
| M1 motorway – the northern route! | North is 'up' – like the brain! |

# Applied mnemonics – the actions of atropine

Now you know the actions of the parasympathetic system you can work out most of the actions of atropine which is a **muscarinic blocker**.

Starting with the CNS with all those M1 (northern route) receptors atropine is excitatory. Not surprisingly as atropine was used to make women appear more beautiful (bella donnas) when they took the stuff (from the deadly nightshade plant *Atropa belladonna*) because it dilated their pupils – muscarinic receptors constrict the pupils. Remember C.C.C.P. – Constriction of Circular muscle opens up the Canal of Schlemm Parasympathetically. So if you block it, the pupils widen.

Moving onto the **heart** we know M2 slow the heart so if atropine blocks this action (of the vagus nerve) the heart will...speed up leaving the beta-1 receptors working just fine and without any opposite slowing down effect of the parasymapathetics.

This brings us to the **lungs**. If the parasympathetic system constricts things then blocking it should help here – and so we have **ipratropium**, derived from atropine (as the name suggests) as a cholinergic muscarinic receptor blocker – used as an inhaler in asthma and chronic airflow limitation to assist breathing.

Now to the **GI** side of things. If M receptors predominantly increase gastric and bladder motility then if we block this effect with atropine maybe it will slow down diarrhoea? Enter co-phenotrope, said to be especially formulated to reduce gut motility for the troops in Vietnam (trade name Lomotil), which contains our buddy atropine.

Stimulating M3 makes you pee – so atropine should have the opposite effect and reduce bladder contractions. Thus, anticholinergics are used to stabilize the bladder and treat incontinence.

**HOT HINT:** Using the same process as above, and working head downwards extrapolate the actions of drugs on the various organ systems.

# NANC transmitters

The NANC (non-adrenergic non-cholinergic) neurotransmitters include nitrous oxide (NO) and the catecholamine dopamine.

### Nancy Boys Are No Dopes

| | |
|---|---|
| **NANC**y boys are | **Non-Adrenergic Non-Cholinergics** |
| **NO** | **Nitrous Oxide** |
| **DOP**es | **Dop**amine |

# Catecholamines

The three stages of **noradrenaline (norepinephrine) synthesis** are: tyrosine → DOPA (dihydroxy-L-phenylalanine) → dopamine → norepinephrine. Although it's a bit outdated now, here's a handy reminder:

### Tired Dopes Do Nada

| | |
|---|---|
| **Tired** | **Tyrosine** |
| **Dopes** | **DOPA** |
| **Do** | **Do**pamine |
| **Nada** | **Noradrenaline** |

## *Alternative*

**Tiresome Dopes Dominate Norway.**

The **enzymes** involved in these three steps are hydroxylase, decarboxylase, and beta-hydroxylase. If the hydroxyl component is represented by the chemical formula (OH) you can use this to remind you:

### Hide De Ho

| | |
|---|---|
| **HiDe** | **Hydroxylase** |
| **De** | **Decarboxylase** |
| **HO** | **Beta-OH-lase (hydroxylase)** |

**Catecholamine metabolism** is via a *cytoplasmic* enzyme called catechol-O-methyltransferase (or COMT) and two *mitochondrial* enzymes called monoamine oxidase A and monoamine oxidase B – the MAOs. Think:

| | |
|---|---|
| **Cytoplasm** | **COMT** |
| **Mitochondria** | **MAO** |

# Zero-order kinetics

It is useful to know some drugs with zero-order kinetics.

### Constantly Aspiring To Phone Ethan

| | |
|---|---|
| **Constantly** | **(zero-order kinetics)** |
| **Aspiring** | **Aspirin** |
| **To PHone** | **Phenytoin** |
| **ETHan** | **Ethanol** |

# 4.2 PHARMACOLOGY AND THERAPEUTICS

## Atorvastatin

**Statins** are generally given only at night because cholesterol synthesis is at its highest overnight. Atorvastatin is the only statin that can be taken at any time because of its long duration of action. Remember it like this:

### At or any time

**At Or**      **Ator**vastatin
**any time**   **day or night**

## Curare

Curare is a competitive inhibitor which blocks nicotinic receptors. Simply put:

**Curare = Competitive inhibitor**

## Loop diuretics

**Furosemide** and **bumetanide** are both loop diuretics. The **loop** of Henle is **U-shaped** like the letter they both share (U) then this is a helpful reminder.

### U-shape (loop of Henle)

**FUrosemide**
**bUmetanide**

## Prostaglandins

**Prostaglandin-1** and **prostaglandin-2** are vasodilators, with their main effects on *arteries*. **Prostaglandin-A** and **prostaglandin-E** are vasodilators, with their main effects on *veins*.

Again substituting the digit '1' with the letter 'I' means you can think of:

*DIlAtE*

**DI**      **1/2**
**LATE**    **A/E**

# The structure of 6 aminopenicillamic acid

6-APA – the basis of the penicillins!

1. Draw a house:

2. Add a garage and smoke from the chimney:

3. Add an outdoor aerial and a garden fence:

4. Stick on an amide group:

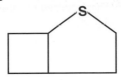

Congratulations!

# Antiepileptics

Current treatment of **petit mal epilepsy** involves use of **valproate** and **ethosuximide**. According to the observation of the 'paradoxical Ps' if a drug name starts with a **P** then it ain't used for **P**etit mal epilepsy!

## Paradoxical Ps

*NOT* for **P**etit mal:
**P**henytoin
**P**rimidone
**P**henobarbital

 **SWOT BOX**

**Petit mal**, or absence seizures, are brief, generalized seizures. They have a particular spike-wave pattern of about 3 Hz on EEG. They usually occur in children aged 4–12 and are characterized by lapses of concentration and rhythmic movements of eyelids and hands. There is rapid return to full consciousness without retrograde amnesia or confusion. Many patients later develop generalized tonic–clonic seizures.

The names of **antiepileptic drugs** are interesting. **Phenytoin** is one of the barbiturates, named after a waitress in Munich called *Barbara* as well as *urea* (according to Sharpless,[1] Barbara even supplied some of the raw materials required). The antiepileptic **vigabatrin** was named after its mode of action, that is inhibition of gamma-aminobutyric acid (GABA)-transferase. The anticonvulsant drug **clobazam** has a name that sounds like the action of knocking patients out (say it quickly!). The analgesic **dolobid** derives from *dolor* (pain of inflammation) and the abbreviation for a twice daily dose *bid*. **Lasix** is furosemide, and it was named thus because it 'lasts six hours'.

# Sympathomimetic amines

Directly acting sympathomimetic amines can be recalled using the mnemonic: I Saw Ape Naked.

### I Saw Ape Naked

**I S**aw **IS**oprenaline
**APE** **EP**inephrine
**N**aked **N**or**A**drenaline (or **N**or**E**pinephrine)

1 Sharpless SK (1965) The barbiturates. In: *The Pharmacological Basis of Therapeutics*, 3rd edn. New York: Macmillan, pp. 105–28.

## *Alternatives*

Try this one: I Saw Adrian Naked (where Adrian stands for adrenaline). Or: Directly I-saw Ape Naked and Acted Sympathetically.

# Antituberculosis drugs

This consists of triple or quadruple therapy – RIP or RIP(E).

### RIP(E)

| | |
|---|---|
| **R** | **Rifampicin** |
| **I** | **Isoniazid** |
| **P** | **Pyrazinamide** |
| **(E)** | **(Ethambutol)** |

Poor compliance to this therapy is best reduced by using combination tablets (such as rifampicin + isoniazid), urine testing for rifampicin (*Prescriber's Journal* 2000: 40(1)) as well as by DOT:

### DOT

| | |
|---|---|
| **D** | **Directly** |
| **O** | **Observed** |
| **T** | **Treatment** |

 SWOT BOX

The **usual regimen** consists of minimum 2 months of RIPE followed by another 4 months of rifampicin + isoniazid (in adults, children, pregnant and breastfeeding women). Depending on the results of cultures, it may be necessary to increase either one or both phases of treatment.

With **CNS involvement** the full course is usually longer (2 months RIPE + 8 months rifampicin + isoniazid).

**HIV patients** are usually given the standard regimen, unless there is multidrug-resistant disease. Liver p450 enzyme induction by rifampicin may make protease inhibitors ineffective, so an alternative retroviral or anti-TB regimen may have to be used.

The **peripheral neuropathy of isoniazid** may be prevented in those at risk (e.g. in HIV, diabetics, chronic renal failure, malnutrition) with 10 mg daily of vitamin B6.

# Beta blockers

This is your first session with spatial mnemonics, covered in much more detail in Section III. We shall use them to learn about beta blockers.

Spatial mnemonics are a little more advanced than simple mnemonics. Such 'spatial' or 'loci' learning systems involve linking something you *need to learn* fast to something *you already know* now – in this case your own body!

Use exaggerated link-association as described in Section III. The *very act* of reading the whole story that follows will help you.

A good system is to start at the head (the CNS) and work downwards. We will use propanolol as our 'typical' beta-blocker. Remember to make your mental images bold, multisensory and exaggerated.

Now if you are up for it, let's roll…

## Effects of propanolol

| CENTRAL NERVOUS SYSTEM | **Propanolol** causes fatigue and depression | *Imagine you are feeling really wonderful and energetic and a 'pro' tries to block this by 'interacting' with your head (brain)* |
|---|---|---|
| EYES | Dilates pupils by blocking the sympa-thetic system so the parasympathetic takes over (e.g. **tim**olol eye drops treat open-angle glaucoma | *If you know somebody called Tim, imagine him putting drops in your eyes* |
| HEART | Blocks beta-1 receptors so the heart slows down as the parasympathetic system takes over (remember, *the vagus nerve (M2) slows the heart, dude*) | *You might think of a heart-stopping heart-throb called Brad, for example* |
| PERIPHERAL VASCULAR SYSTEM | Vasoconstriction. Remember *beta makes 'em bigger*. Well, if you block this, then the opposite happens, resulting in **freezing** cold extremities | *'Brrrr…Brr…Brad!'* |

| | | |
|---|---|---|
| **LUNGS** | **Broncho**constriction beta-2 effect (remember, *2 lungs*) | *Imagine something like a wheezing bucking **bronco** on your chest* |
| **MUSCULOSKELETAL** | Reduces tremor | *That **pro** is calming things down* |
| **METABOLIC** | Raises cholesterol | *Hey, you do some work here!* |
| **KINETICS** | It is protein bound with a short half-life of 4 hours | |

Once you have a spatial sequence to your liking, pencil it down and work through it a few times in your head. You will find that you will remember much more material this way, and it is significantly quicker to review the night before your exam. You can use any well-known objects, structures and people with this technique, like your own house for alpha-blockers, your porch for penicillin, and your kitchen for the Krebs cycle!

# Chapter Five

# MICROBIOLOGY AND INFECTIOUS DISEASES

*When you have read this chapter you will be able to tackle the following with ease:*

---

## ? PRE-QUIZ

1 What are the complications of mumps?
2 Is *Neisseria* a Gram-negative or Gram-positive organism?
3 Does *Shigella* have flagella for motility?
4 Can you name some non-lactose fermenters?
5 What are the features of syphilis?

---

## Diarrhoea in kids

Endemic **viral diarrhoea** in children is predominantly associated with rotaviruses, adenoviruses, caliciviruses and astroviruses. These are represented by:

### Aiden strokes Cali's rottweiler

| | |
|---|---|
| **Aiden** | **Aden**oviruses |
| **Stro**kes | a**Stro**viruses |
| **Cali**'s | **Cali**civiruses |
| **Rot**tweiler | **Rot**aviruses |

# Mumps

Moping about mumps is a sure-fire way of remembering its four main symptoms.

## MOPE

| | |
|---|---|
| **M** | **Meningism** |
| **O** | **Orchitis/Oophoritis** |
| **P** | **Parotitis/Pancreatitis/Paramyxovirus** |
| **E** | **Encephalitis** |

### SWOT BOX

Mumps is an air-borne **paramyxovirus** (it is also spread by direct contact with body fluids). Uncommon in adults, it is often subclinical in children. Usually salivary gland inflammation is the principal manifestation (e.g. uni- or bilateral parotitis).

**Complications** include epididymo-orchitis, oophoritis, meningo-encephalitis and pancreatitis. Mumps meningitis is usually benign, with vomiting, neck rigidity, lethargy, headache, photophobia, convulsions, and abdominal pain and fever.

# *Neisseria* – negative sugar

Microbiologists use cultures containing glucose and maltose to differentiate between the negative cocci *Neisseria meningitides* and *Neisseria gonorrhoea*. This is called the sugar fermentation test. *Neisseria gonorrhoea* ferments glucose only, while *Neisseria meningitides* ferments glucose and maltose.

| | |
|---|---|
| ***N. gonorrhoea*** | **Ferments glucose only** |
| ***N. meningitides*** | **Ferments maltose as well** |

# RNA viruses

It might only be a coincidence, but most RNA viruses start with the letter '**R**' – like **r**habdovirus, **r**eovirus, **r**otavirus, and **r**hinovirus. Yet another coincidence is that drugs containing the letters '**vir**' are often anti**vir**al – like Retro**vir**, Zo**vir**ax and Vecta**vir**. So in general:

| RNA viruses | Start with the letter **R** |
|---|---|
| Anti**VIR**al drugs | Contain the letters **VIR** |

# *Salmonella* and *Shigella*

Both these organisms are important in food poisoning. They are both non-lactose fermenters. *Salmonella* are flagellate organisms and are motile, whilst *Shigella* have no flagella and are therefore non-motile. But can you remember which one is the motile one when you are under pressure? Well you can easily – if you think of a salmon and remember that it is motile – so is *Salmonella*!

### *Salmonella* are motile like **salmon**

Try drawing a picture of a salmon(ella).

You can learn all the **non-lactose fermenters** with **SSPP**.

### SSPP

| S | Salmonella |
|---|---|
| S | Shigella |
| P | Pseudomonas |
| P | Proteus |

# Cytomegalovirus

The abbreviation for cytomegalovirus is CMV, which – somewhat conveniently – is an acronym for the main symptoms of the disease.

### CMV

| C | Colitis |
|---|---|
| M | Mouth dysphagia and oesophogeal ulceration |
| V | Visual problems (retinitis) |

# Syphilis

Syphilis is a subacute to chronic infectious disease caused by the spirochete *Treponema pallidum.* Doctors used to treat it with *quacksalver*, a cream containing mercury. The word *quack* derives from this. Quacksalver became *quicksilver* which is still a synonym for the element mercury. A popular joke when this disease hit Europe was 'You spend one night with Venus – and six months with Mercury'!

A small red papule or crusted erosion called a **chancre** appears at the site of inoculation as a painless primary lesion, which often breaks down with a serous exudate. The tertiary stage occurs after many years, as neurosyphilis, with neurological symptoms that include **tabes dorsalis** and **delusions of grandeur**. Tabes in neurosyphilis is a progressive degeneration of the posterior columns, posterior roots and ganglia of the spinal cord, giving symptoms such as lightning pains, ataxia, urinary incontinence, optic atrophy, Charcot's joints, hypotonia and hyper-reflexia. Transmission may also be *in utero* (see TORCHS on p. 122), leading to various congenital manifestations, including anterior bowing of the mid-portion of the tibia (**sabre shin**). This is a late congenital sign, seen less frequently now due to treatment with penicillin.

Here is a great summary of what the condition involves:[1]

**There was a young lad from Bombay**
**Whose chancre just wouldn't fade away**
**Well, apart from his tabes**
**and sabre-legged babies**
**Now he thinks he's Fay Wray!**

 **SWOT BOX**

Syphilis was the name of a shepherd infected with the disease in a poem of Fracastorius (1530), perhaps derived from the Greek *syn* (together) and *philein* (to love). It appeared in Europe at the siege of Naples (1495). As it spread through the continent, the French called it the Italian disease, the Italians called it the Spanish disease, and the Spanish called it the English disease...[2,3]

Another symptom classically associated with syphilis (which also occurs in conditions such as diabetes and Wernicke's encephalopathy) is the Argyll Robertson pupil. This is named after Douglas Moray Cooper Lamb Argyll Robertson (1837–1909) who was President of the College of Surgeons of Edinburgh in 1886.

---

1 Contributed by Dr Bobby Bhartia, SGUL.
2 From Gertz SD, Gaithersburg MD (1996) *Liebman's Neuroanatomy Made Easy and Understandable*, 3rd edn. Aspen Publishers and *Dorling's Medical Dictionary*, 28th edn. Philadelphia: WB Saunders.
3 Kirstin Harper (Emory University, Atlanta, USA, 2008) has described how syphilis may have originated in South America (Columbus returned from the New World in 1492).

**NAUGHTY BIT**

Why is an Argyll Robertson pupil like a prostitute?
*Because it accommodates but doesn't react!*

# Tuberculosis

 **RAPID REVISION**

Therapy of TB was discussed on p. 55. Initial treatment is with triple or quadruple therapy – with RIP or RIP(E) – with Rifampicin, Isoniazid, Pyrazinamide (and Ethambutol). Further treatment is with just rifampicin and isoniazid. Patient compliance can be problem.

# SECTION II

## CLINICAL SPECIALTIES

# Chapter Six

# CHEMICAL PATHOLOGY

*The physician…has to know the cause of the ailment before he can cure it*
Mocius (c.470–390 BC)

*By time you've mused through this section you will be able to tackle these:*

> ## ? PRE-QUIZ
>
> 1 How many causes of a low plasma sodium can you think of?
> 2 Can you think of any causes of a raised potassium?
> 3 Can you list three causes of lowered serum phosphate?
> 4 What does a low plasma T4 level with a low level of thyroid-stimulating hormone suggest?
> 5 What about a low plasma T4 and a high thyroid-stimulating hormone level?
> 6 What are the features of Conn's syndrome?

## Addison's disease

Addison's is the syndrome of adrenal insufficiency. To remind yourself of this, look carefully at the name Addison's.

### Adrenal is No' Sufficient

**ADDISON'S    AD**renal **IS NO,** Sufficient

# Raised alkaline phosphatase

### Plate of Liver and Kidney Beans

| | |
|---|---|
| **Plate of** | **Placental alkaline phosphatase in pregnancy** |
| **Liver and** | **Liver disease (?cholestasis)** |
| **Kidney** | **Renal failure** |
| **Beans** | **Bone disease (*isoenzyme*)** |

The isoenzyme is related to osteoblast activity, especially in Paget's disease, child growth, healing, metastases, osteomalacia and hyperparathyroidism.

# Bilirubin – unconjugated

Remember the causes with this simple memory jogger.

### Uncle Gilbert's Creaky Home

| | |
|---|---|
| **Unc**le | **Unc**onjugated due to... |
| **Gilbert's** | **Gilbert's** |
| **Cr**eaky | **Cr**igler–Najjar |
| **H**ome | **H**aemolysis |

# Conn's syndrome

The important features of Conn's are low renin, high aldosterone, alkalosis, low potassium and hypertension, and common presentations are high blood pressure, fatigue, muscle pain and headaches. The syndrome is name after J.W. Conn, a US physician. Here is a good ditty for getting these main features into your memory.

| | |
|---|---|
| An **alkalotic** young **CON**man named Mervin | **Alkalosis, Con**n's syndrome |
| Had headache 'cos there was **no rainin'** | **Headaches No renin** |
| With no **pot** to grow | Low **pot**assium |
| A lot of **pressure**, you know | High blood **pressure** |
| **High aldosterone** was making him **paining**! | **High aldosterone** and **muscle cramps** |

# Plasma phosphate

Causes of **raised plasma phosphate** are renal failure, delayed separation of sample and vitamin D excess. Here is a mnemonic for you to try.

### It's Rough Waiting With VD

| It's Rough | **Renal failure** |
| **Waiting** with | **(delayed** separation) |
| **VD** | **Vitamin D** |

Add 'Fanny' to the above to remind you of 'phosphate' – if you think it's necessary, as in 'It's Rough Waiting With VD, Fanny'.

Causes of **low phosphate** are high parathyroid hormone (PTH), low vitamin D and hypoventilation.

### Lowly Phil Ate Dee's Breathless Parrot

| **Lowly Phil** ate | **Low Ph**osphate |
| **Dee's** | **Vitamin D (low)** |
| **Breathless** | **Hypoventilation** |
| **Parrot** | **PTH (high)** |

# Raised potassium

What's behind raised potassium levels?

### Too Much Pot Delayed Milo – Now Him Frigid

| **Too much pot** | Hyperkalaemia |
| **Delays** | **Delay**ed separation of sample/difficult venesection |
| **Milo** | **Myelo**proliferative disorders |
| **NOW** | **NOW** take biochemistry samples, before any others! |
| **Him** | **Haemolysis** |
| **Frig**id | **Frig**de (for storing blood) |

# Hyponatraemia

For the causes of low plasma sodium, use this memorable phrase.

### Adding Sid's Hair Dye Creates Seriously Low Volume

| | |
|---|---|
| **Add**ing | **Add**ison's |
| **Sid**'s | **SIAD**H (syndrome of inappropriate ADH) |
| **H**air | **H**ypothyroid |
| **D**ye | **D**iuretics (especially thiazides) |
| **C**reates | **C**arbamazepine |
| **S**eriously | **SS**RIs (selective serotonin reuptake inhibitors) |
| Low **volume** | **Volume** depreciation (postural drop in blood pressure) |

# Thyroid hormones

A **low serum free T4** level alone could mean an underactive thyroid or pituitary gland failure. Therefore we need to look at the thyroid-stimulating hormone (TSH) level also. A **high TSH level** would confirm that the thyroid gland (not the pituitary gland) is responsible for the hypothyroidism. An underactive **'lazy' thyroid** gland gives us a **low T4 and a high TSH** – where the pituitary is 'flogging' the gland to get it to produce more thyroxine.

So think of:

### Hitesh's Letter To Lazy Gland

| | |
|---|---|
| **Hitesh's** | **Hi TSH** |
| **Letter To** | **Low T4** |
| **Lazy gland** | **Lazy thyroid gland** |

The usual cause of the pituitary gland failure is tumour.

So think:

### Trish and Terrier Fell in Pit

| | |
|---|---|
| **Tri**SH | Low **TSH** |
| **and** | + |
| **T**errier | **T4** |
| **Fell** in | **Falling** levels = |
| **Pit** | **Pit**uitary problem |

To sum it all up:

**Low** T4   +   **High** TSH   =   Lazy **Thyroid**
**Low** T4   +   **Low** TSH   =   Failed **Pituitary**

 **SWOT BOX**

A failing pituitary gland that is not producing TSH is not stimulating the thyroid to produce T4. Since the pituitary gland also regulates other glands (adrenals, gonads) as well as controlling growth and normal kidney function, failure means that the other glands may also be underactive.

*Medicine is an art and attends to the nature of the (individual) patient and has principles of action and reason in each case*
Plato (*Symposium*)

# Chapter Seven

# MEDICAL SPECIALTIES

*This chapter spans general medicine, cardiovascular and chest medicine, dermatology, endocrinology, gastroenterology, haematology, neurology, renal medicine and urology. As you read and learn about the subjects covered here you will be able to answer all the following, and more:*

## ? PRE-QUIZ

1 What does CREST stand for in CREST syndrome?
2 Can you list the features of acromegaly?
3 What are the features associated with carcinoid syndrome?
4 What are the X-ray features of Crohn's?
5 Which amino acids are not reabsorbed in cystinuria?
6 How would you manage diabetic ketoacidosis?
7 Can you name at least six causes of clubbing?
8 What are the ECG features of low potassium?
9 What are the six main types of exudate?
10 What are the risk factors for congenital dislocation of the hip?
11 Which pain fibres carry crude touch sensations?
12 Which nerve roots are affected if there is an absent biceps jerk reflex?
13 What are the main causes of mononeuritis multiplex?
14 What are the signs of a cerebellar lesion?

# 7.1 GENERAL MEDICINE AND PATHOLOGY

## Clubbing

Clubbing consists of loss of nail-bed angle, increased curvature of the nail (sideways and lengthways) and increased sponginess of the nail bed. The causes of clubbing are numerous. You can easily remember them when they are grouped like this:

### The 8 Cs of Clubbing[1]

| | |
|---|---|
| Carcinoma | **Such as lung carcinoma or stomach carcinoma** |
| Cardiac | **Such as bacterial endocarditis or cyanotic congenital heart disease** |
| Cervical rib | **Causing neurovascular compression in the upper limb** |
| Chest | **Such as cystic fibrosis, empyema, bronchiectasis, tuberculosis (with extensive fibrosis), fibrosing alveolitis or abscess of lung** |
| Circulation | **Such as atrioventricular (AV) fistula in arm (kidney dialysis patients)** |
| Cirrhosis | **Of the liver (check for other signs of liver disease)** |
| Colonic | **Such as Crohn's, ulcerative colitis and coeliac disease** |
| Congenital | |

And here is an easy way to check for clubbing, known as the **'diamond' sign**. Put your thumbs together, back-to-back, with the thumbnails facing and touching each other. With normal nails you can see a thin diamond-shaped gap from the top of the knuckle to the top of the nail. This 'diamond' is not seen with clubbing of the nails. If you draw this for yourself now you are unlikely to forget it – the physical act will reinforce the memory.

1 This version is after A. Ala.

## SWOT BOX

Cervical ribs occur in 1% of the population, where embryological cervical elements form cervical ribs from C7. These may impinge on the subclavian artery and inferior trunk of the brachial plexus, resulting in neurovascular compression syndrome of the upper limb.

Carcinoid tumours are neuroendocrine in origin and produce a variety of different polypeptide hormones and products, especially serotonin (5-HT). Tumours are generally in the gastrointestinal tract and are often asymptomatic. Carcinoid syndrome (below) is usually associated with ileal carcinoids because hepatic decarboxylation is avoided.

Pseudo-clubbing occurs in thyroid disease.

And yet more on clubbing...

### CLUB'D

| | |
|---|---|
| **C** | **Cyanotic heart disease; Crohn's disease** |
| **L** | **Lung disease; liver disease** |
| **U** | **Ulcerative colitis** |
| **B** | **Bacterial endocarditis** |
| **D** | **Diarrhoea (chronic)** |

# Crest syndrome

Here is a 'spatial' mnemonic for Crest syndrome, to remind you what it consists of. We can use a spatial mnemonics to learn this as there are five things we can easily link to the five digits of our own hand using exaggerated (and ridiculous) mental associations. Look at each digit in turn and picture as vividly as you can the following descriptions.

| Symptom | Which digit | What to imagine as you look |
|---|---|---|
| Calcinosis | Thumb | Whoa! It's become completely calcified! |
| Raynaud's phenomenon | Index finger | It's bright blue and so cold! |
| Oesophogeal dysmotility | Middle finger | Imagine sticking it down your throat like an endoscope |

| Sclerodactyly | Ring finger | Lots of tight rings that won't come off – so tight at the top of your finger that it's becoming tapered |
| Telangiectasia | Little finger | Hold it to your ear like a telephone (that's a 'substitute word' for telangiectasia) |

 **SWOT BOX**

**Calcinosis** is seen as palpable nodules in the hands due to calcific deposits in subcutaneous tissues.

**Sclerodactyly** is tightening of the skin of the hand, that leads to tapering of the fingers.

**Telangiectasia** in Crest syndrome are multiple and large, and present on the hands.

For more on spatial mnemonics see Section III.

# Dupuytren's contracture

Dupuytren's is a fibrous contracture of the palmar fascia. You need to know the causes.

### Alcoholic Doctors Fit a History of Trauma

| | |
|---|---|
| **Alcoholic** | **Alcohol** |
| **Doctors** | **Diabetes mellitus** |
| **Fit** a | **Fits** (as with epilepsy) |
| **History** of | **History** (family) |
| **Trauma** | **Trauma** (repeated, of the hand as in manual workers) |

## *Alternative*

You can add 'doped' to remind you of 'Dupuytren's' to make: Doped Alcoholic Doctors Fit a History of Trauma.

**SWOT BOX**

Baron Dupuytren (1777–1835) has a fascinating biography. He was kidnapped at the age of four by a wealthy lady (he was said to be a very attractive child) and later returned. He went to medical school in Paris and at age eighteen was in charge of all the post mortems. We hear he was a very difficult person to get on with, perhaps due to this early trauma. He had early financial difficulties but ended up very wealthy, having built up a substantial practice. He suffered a stroke while lecturing in 1833 and died a few months later.

# Exudates

An exudate is material that has escaped from blood vessels or tissues and is characterized by a high protein content. This mnemonic covers all the different types of exudate you need to know about.

### Ham, sir? Remember Cats Prefer Fish

| | |
|---|---|
| **Ham** | **Haemorrhagic** |
| **Sir** | **Serous** |
| **Remember** | **Membranous** |
| **Cats** | **Catarrhal** |
| **Prefer** | **Purulent** |
| **Fish** | **Fibrinous** |

# HLA-B27

Conditions associated with the **human leukocyte antigen** HLA-B27:

### Hillbillies colliding sore ankles are irate

| | |
|---|---|
| **HiLlBillies** | **HLA-B27** |
| **Colliding** | **Colitis** |
| **Sore** | **Psoriasis** |
| **AnkleS** | **Ankylosing Spondylitis** |
| **are (R)** | **Reiter's** |
| **Irate** | **Iritis (with the Reiter's)** |

# Immunoglobulins

 **RAPID REVISION**

We have already seen on p. 42 that the five classes if Ig are GAMED.

Ig M is produced first in the primary immune response (it is produced IMmediately). IgG appears as the IgM level falls, forming the **secondary** response, which is due to activation of long-lived B cells on repeat exposure to the antigen.

# Bone metabolism

Osteo*blasts build* the bone and osteo*clasts cut* it away.

| | |
|---|---|
| **Blasts** | **Build** |
| **Clasts** | **Cut away** |

# Rashes and fevers

The following anonymous chart is a guide to which day the rash typically appears on after the prodrome – e.g. the rubella rash develops on the first day of the onset of fever/illness, and the scarlet fever rash appears on the second day. Note there is no rash appearing at day 6.

### Really Sick People Must Take No Exercise

| **Really** | **Rubella** | **Day 1** |
|---|---|---|
| **Sick** | **Scarletina** | **Day 2** |
| **People** | **smallPox** | **Day 3** |
| **Must** | **Measles** | **Day 4** |
| **Take** | **Typhoid fever** | **Day 5** |
| **No** | **(none)** | **Day 6** |
| **Exercise** | **Enteric fever** | **Day 7** |

# Rheumatic fever

The five major (Jones') criteria for **acute** rheumatic fever are carditis (40 per cent), erythema marginatum (10–60 per cent), subcutaneous nodules (10 per cent), arthritis (migratory large-joint polyarthritis; 90 per cent) and Sydenham's chorea (rapid, involuntary, purposeless and jerky movements, from Latin *chorea*; Greek *choreia*, meaning to dance). Some people use the mnemonic CHANCE, but even better than this is 'Arthur's Red Cardigan'.

## Noodles and Curry On Arthur's Red Cardigan

| Noodles and | Nodules |
| --- | --- |
| Curry on | Chorea |
| Arthur's | Arthritis |
| Red | Erythema |
| Cardigan | Carditis |

 **SWOT BOX**

The **acute** systemic illness is due to infection by a beta-haemolytic *Streptococcus*, usually between the ages of 5 and 15 years. The heart and joints are mainly affected. There may be myo-, endo- or pericarditis.

The minor criteria are **fe**ver, **a**rthralgia and **r**aised white cell count (**FeAR**). Confirmation of streptococcal infection and two major criteria are diagnostic (or one major and two minor).

If the attack is severe or occurs in early childhood or is recurrent, the disease may progress to chronic rheumatic heart disease (RHD). It is suggested that there is cross-reactivity between streptococcal and cardiac antigens. Chronic RHD is the largest global cause of heart disease, although it is less common in developed countries, probably due to the use of antibiotics (the streptococci are susceptible to penicillin).

# Rheumatoid arthritis

This tells you the hand deformities in rheumatoid arthritis.

## BUS'Z

| B | Boutonniére |
| --- | --- |
| U | Ulnar deviation |
| S | Swan neck |
| Z | Z deformity (thumb) |

It is also possible to see triggering of the finger (flexor tendon nodule) as well as erythema of the palms (which gives us BUSZ-TE).

# Shock

These are the different types.

### CASHED

| | |
|---|---|
| **C** | **Cardiac** |
| **A** | **Anaphylactic** |
| **S** | **Septic** |
| **H** | **Hypovolaemic** |
| **E** | **Endocrine (e.g. Addison's)** |
| **D** | **Drugs (e.g. anaesthetics)** |

# Syphilis

 **RAPID REVISION**

This has already been covered (pages 61 and 62) but can you remember the stages and characteristics of syphilis? Do you recall that young lad from Bombay?

# Vitamin D deficiency

Polly can help you remember the main features of this vitamin deficiency.

### Polly Is Only A Shilling

| | |
|---|---|
| **Polly** | **Pernicious anaemia** |
| **Is** | **Intrinsic factor (lack of)** |
| **Only** | **Only confirmed if B12 deficiency is due to pernicious anaemia** |
| **A** | **Antibodies vs parietal cells** |
| **Shilling** | **Schilling test** |

 **SWOT BOX**

The **Schilling test** checks that the vitamin B12 deficiency is due to pernicious anaemia – which is correctable by giving **intrinsic factor**. In the test, parenteral radiolabelled B12 is given with oral B12. A 24-hour urine demonstrates that oral B12 is not absorbed. The test is then with swallowed capsules of intrinsic factor – this corrects the deficiency due to pernicious anaemia *only*.

## 7.2 CARDIOLOGY

# Aortic stenosis

For the main features, remember:

### Middle-Aged Men Force Thrills Slowly

| | |
|---|---|
| **Middle**-aged **Men** | **Mid**-systolic **Murmur** |
| **Force** | **Force**ful apex beat |
| **Thrills** | systolic **Thrill** (at base of heart) |
| **Slowly** | **Slow** rising pulse |

# Atrial fibrillation

The three types of atrial fibrillation can be classified as PERsistent, PARoxysmal or PERManent – that is, three Ps. Yet despite so many Ps, atrial fibrillation is characterized by a lack of P waves on the ECG! Which gives us:

### 3 Ps – But no 'p' on ECG!

## *Alternative*

PERcy's PARrot's PERM.

# Bundle branch block

What happens to the shape of the ECG when there is a bundle branch block?

With a **right branch block** there is an M-shaped wave in V1, and sometimes a W-shaped wave in V6. To remember this, think of a marrow:

### MARROW

| | |
|---|---|
| Ma | V1 |
| **RRo** | **(right** bundle branch block) |
| W | V6 |

With a **left branch block** you get a W-shaped complex in V1 and occasionally an M-shaped complex in V6. Thanks to William we get:

## WILLIAM

| Wi | V1 |
|---|---|
| **LL**ia | (**left** bundle branch block) |
| M | V6 |

# Cardiac troponins

There are three types of troponins – C, T and I. Troponins C and I are the cardiac ones. They are very sensitive indicators of cardiac damage, but they are not too specific, so this rule of Cs will help you to know the other six major causes of raised cardiac troponins.

### The C Rule

| **Cardiac** arrest | **myocardial infarction** |
|---|---|
| **Cardiac** failure | **severe heart failure** |
| **Cocaine** | **causes coronary artery spasm** |
| **Carditis** | **myocarditis** |
| **Car** accident | **or some other trauma** |
| **Chest** | **pulmonary emboli** |

 **SWOT BOX**

Cardiac troponins are released from striated muscles cells within 12 hours of cardiac damage. They are present for several days after the event.

# Central cyanosis

The causes of central cyanosis are made quite memorable with this mnemonic.

### Tense Fresher's Cope Emphasizing Arty 'Pnemonics'!

| **T**ense | **Tension pneumothorax** |
|---|---|
| **Fresher's** | **Fibrosing alveolitis** |
| **Cope** | **COPD** |
| **Emph**asizing | **Emph**ysema |
| **A**rty | **A**sthma |
| **Pneum**onics! | **Pneum**onia |

# Coarctation of the aorta

The natural history of aortic coarctation involves hypertension, heart failure, aortic aneurysm rupture, endocarditis, and aortic valve disease (regurgitation, stenosis, biscuspid valves). To remind yourself of these important features you could think of:

### Hyperactive Avril Oughta Fail Endo

| | |
|---|---|
| **Hyperactive** | **Hypertension** |
| **AVRil** | **Aortic Valve disease (including Regurgitation, AVR)** |
| **Oughta** | **Aorta (rhymes) (aneurysm rupture)** |
| **Fail** | heart **Failure** |
| **Endo** | **Endo**carditis |

# Congestive cardiac failure

Left ventricular failure (LVF) manifests as acute difficulty in breathing, while right heart failure (RVF) tends to cause swellings in peripheral areas and is particularly evident in the lower limbs. Think:

**L** VF affects the **Lungs**
**R** VF affects the **Rest (leading to fluid overload)**

# Right ventricular failure – fluid overload

Here is a useful way to remember the signs of fluid overload.

### Fat Ella Jumps and Gallops Over Livid Plums

| | |
|---|---|
| **Fat** | **Fat**igue |
| **Ella Jumps and** | **Elevated JVP** |
| **Gallops** | **Gallop** rhythm – S3 heart sound |
| **Over** | **O**edema |
| **Livid** | **Liv**er enlarged |
| **Plums** | **P**leural effusion |

# ECG leads

Connecting up the ECG leads is easy when you think of some traffic lights – they have to be broken ones so they end in 'black'. Start *clockwise* from the right side of the patient:

### Traffic lights

| | |
|---|---|
| Red | **Right** arm |
| Yellow | Left arm |
| Green | Left leg |
| Black | Right leg |

## *Alternative*

### Read Your Good Book, *or* Ride Your Green Bike.

Why don't you reinforce this by sketching a DaVinci-style body on a clock face with all four limbs stretching out to the edge of the clock?

**Heart rate** is determined from the big squares on the ECG trace like this:

| Number of big squares | Heart rate (beats per minute) |
|---|---|
| 1 | 300 |
| 2 | 150 |
| 3 | 100 |
| 4 | 75 |
| 5 | 60 |
| 6 | 50 |

# Endocarditis

The main features of endocarditis are given by:

### Splendid Feverish Vegetarians Enjoy Clubbing Till a.m.

| | |
|---|---|
| **Splen**did | **Splen**omegaly |
| **Fever**ishly | **Fever** (> 1 week, > 38.5°C) |
| **Veget**arians | **Veget**ations (on echo) |
| **E**njoy | **E**mboli (come off the vegetations) |
| **Clubbing** | **Clubbing** |
| **T**ill | **T**ricuspid valve (in IV drug abusers) |
| A.M. | **A**ortic and **M**itral valves (usually affected) |

The infecting organisms in endocarditis are shown here.

**Grannie Enjoys Straps and Staples**

| | |
|---|---|
| **Gran**nie | **Gram** negative bacteria |
| **Enjoys** | **E**nterococci |
| **Straps** and | **Strep**tococci |
| **Staples** | **Stap**hylococci |

# Hypertension

The causes of hypertension are made far more memorable with this quick reminder.

**CREEP**

| | |
|---|---|
| **C** | **C**oarctation of the aorta |
| **R** | **R**enal |
| **E** | **E**ndocrine |
| **E** | **E**clampsia (essential) |
| **P** | **P**ill or Phaeocromocytoma |

# Left atrial enlargement (P mitrale)

The ECG of this condition shows a **bifid P wave** (of duration 0.12 seconds or more). The two peaks are due to delayed response from the enlarged left atrium. The first peak is from the right atrium, and the second is from the left. In P mitrale, therefore, the trace looks like a letter 'm', so remember:

**P mitrale looks like letter 'm'**      **(m for mitrale)**

Draw this quickly to reinforce the image in your head.

# Lipoproteins

Here's how to distinguish between good and bad lipoproteins. Very-low-density lipoproteins (VLDLs) carry triglycerides from hepatic to peripheral and other cells, where they are stored and later used for metabolism. High-density lipoproteins (HDLs) carry cholesterol away from the peripheral cells to the liver for excretion. Therefore, you can think of them as:

**H (for HDL) are Heroes**
**V (for VLDL) are Villains**

# Low plasma potassium

When plasma potassium drops, the shape of the ECG changes, the height of the T wave becomes flattened. Thus, you should remember:

**No Pot – No Tea!**

# Mitral stenosis

According to Rubenstein and Wayne,[1] the development of pulmonary hypertension in mitral stenosis is indicated by APRIL.

### APRIL

| | |
|---|---|
| **A** | **A dominant 'a' wave of the jugular venous pulse (unless in atrial fibrillation)** |
| **P** | **Pulmonary valve (second sound is loud)** |
| **R** | **Right ventricular hypertrophy** |
| **I** | **Incompetence (pulmonary – rare)** |
| **L** | **Low peripheral arterial pulse volume** |

# Murmurs and heart sounds

 **RAPID REVISION**

Before we cover systolic and diastolic murmurs, we need a quick reminder about **heart sounds**. On p. 49 we learnt about the Mighty Ape, as a convenient way to relate the mitral (M) and tricuspid (T) components and aortic (A) and pulmonary (P) valve closures.

Diastolic murmurs can be summed up by DAIMS.

### DAIMS

| | |
|---|---|
| **D** | **Diastolic** |
| **AI** | **Aortic Incompetence** |
| **MS** | **Mitral Stenosis** |

And **systolic murmurs** by this phrase:

1 Rubenstein D, Wayne D (2002) *Lecture Notes in Clinical Medicine*. Edinburgh: Blackwells.

**As Innocent Mr Terry Passes VD**

| | |
|---|---|
| **AS** | **Aortic Stenosis** |
| **Innocent** | **Innocent murmur** |
| **MR** | **Mitral Regurgitation (MR)** |
| **TeRry** | **Tricuspid Regurgitation (TR)** |
| **PASSes** | **PulmonAry StenosiS** |
| **VD** | **Ventricular septal Defect** |

# Pericarditis

In pericarditis the ECG trace characteristically shows a 'saddle-shaped' raised ST segment in most leads. You Park Your Car before you get in a saddle.

**Park-your-car**

| | |
|---|---|
| **Park your** | **Peri...** |
| **Car** | **car(ditis)** |

# Prevention of heart disease

Secondary prevention of heart disease after myocardial infarct includes the following:

**ACE–ABC**

| | |
|---|---|
| **ACE** | **ACE inhibitors** |
| **A** | **Aspirin** |
| **B** | **Beta-blocker** |
| **C** | **Calcium-channel blocker** |

# Raynaud's phenomenon

Raynaud's manifests as intermittent ischaemia of the fingers and toes with severe pallor, cyanosis, pain and numbness. WBC gives the colour changes observed in the extremities in Raynaud's, in order.

**Raynaud's WBC**

| | |
|---|---|
| **White** | **Arteriolar spasm** |
| **Blue** | **Dilated capillaries (skin feels cold, numb)** |
| **Crimson red** | **Reactive hyperaemia (as the vasospasm relaxes)** |

**SWOT BOX**

Raynaud was a French physician (1834–1881). His 'phenomenon' was the subject of his thesis. Raynaud's is aggravated by cold or emotional stimuli and relieved by heat, and is secondary to some other abnormality, such as systemic lupus erythematosus (SLE), scleroderma, cervical rib, trauma from vibrating tools, or drugs like beta-blockers, ergotamine, oral oestrogens. When the cause is primary, familial or idiopathic, it is called Raynaud's disease. The latter is more common in women.

**Raynaud's Disease we Don't know**
**Phenomenon has a Pathological cause**

Some of the causes are listed in the chapter on Surgery on p. 132, under the mnemonic: My Servant's Vibrator's So Cold, Ergo Dames Thighs Are Nervous.

# Rheumatic fever

**RAPID REVISION**

You may remember the five major criteria (Jones' criteria) for **acute rheumatic fever,** which are carditis, erythema marginatum, subcutaneous nodules, arthritis and Sydenham's chorea, as specified by the mnemonic 'Noodles and Curry on Arthur's Red Cardigan'. Details are on pp. 75–6.

# Volume depletion

The signs of depletion are conveniently explained by one word – DEPLETE.

**DEPLETE**

| | |
|---|---|
| **D** | **Dry mucous membranes** |
| **E** | **Extremities are cold** |
| **P** | **Pulse faint (postural hypotension)** |
| **L** | **Loss of weight** |
| **E** | **Electrolytes abnormal** |
| **T** | **Tachycardia** |
| **E** | **Elasticity of skin (turgor) is reduced** |

# 7.3 CHEST MEDICINE

## Pleuritic pain

How can you learn all the causes of pleuritic pain? Try this:

### Concert News: Fresher Slips Sucking Paul's Shiny Muscular Pen

| | |
|---|---|
| Concert | Cancer |
| News | Pneumonia |
| Fresher | Fracture |
| Slips | Slipped disc (neuropathic pain) |
| Sucking | Coxsackie virus (Bornholm's) |
| Paul's | Pleurisy |
| Shiny | Shingles |
| Muscular | Musculoskeletal injury |
| PEn | Pulmonary Embolus |

## Haemoptysis

These are the major causes.

### Cancel new tablets – bring crone blood

| | |
|---|---|
| Cancel | Cancer |
| New | Pneumonia |
| Tablets | Tuberculosis |
| Bring | Bronchiectasis |
| Crone | Chronic bronchitis |
| Blood | Blood clot (pulmonary embolism) |

## Respiratory failure

Here are some tips for remembering the features of types 1 and 2 respiratory failure. In both types, oxygen is lost but we measure parameters of oxygen and carbon dioxide. In type 1, oxygen is low (only one parameter is affected). In type 2, both carbon dioxide and oxygen are affected.

| Type | Parameters affected[2] |
|------|------------------------|
| 1 | 1 (oxygen) |
| 2 | 2 (oxygen and carbon dioxide) |

# Stridor and wheeze

*Stridor* is a harsh, grating and frequently high-pitched breath sound; it is almost always inspiratory, produced by upper respiratory obstruction (such as in croup). *Wheezes* are polyphonic, high-pitched sounds, usually caused by intrapulmonary airways obstruction. They are usually expiratory sounds. How do you remember the difference? Simple:

| | |
|---|---|
| **StrIdor** | **InSpIratory** |
| **WhEEzE** | **Expiratory...** |

 **SWOT BOX**

The causes of stridor include laryngotracheobronchitis or croup (mainly parainfluenza type III virus), foreign bodies, *Haemophilus influenzae* type B infection, epiglottitis (or 'supraglottitis'), upper respiratory inflammation (from corrosive/hot/irritant fumes and gases), laryngomalacia (congenital floppy larynx), congenital vascular ring, retropharyngeal abscess, post-intubation, *Corynebacterium diphtheriae* infection (diphtheria), angioedema and tetany and mediastinal masses.

# Tuberculosis

See more about TB treatment in the chapters on Pharmacology and Microbiology.

---

2  Dr Shahid Khan, Consultant Gastroenterologist, St Mary's Hospital, London.

# 7.4 DERMATOLOGY

## Epiloia (tuberous sclerosis)

This is rare (except in textbooks). It is autosomal dominant disorder of skin and central nervous system, diagnosed in childhood. Important clinical features include **shagreen patches**, **subungual fibromas** (smooth, pinkish projections which grow form the nail base), **retinal phakomas** (white streaks along the fundal vessels – epiloia is often classed as a phacomatosis), **adenoma sebaceum** (pinkish papules on facial skin which can be confused with acne) and **ash-leaf macules** (elongated or ovoid hypopigmented macules). It is a cause of learning difficulty. This mnemonic is suitably rude.

> So there was that ol' **shagger** from Bourneville
> Who bit off his **fibromas, subungual**
> 'Oh **phakoma**!' he cried
> 'These **adenomas** won't hide –
> and all these **ash-leaves** just look like a jungle!'

 **SWOT BOX**

This is also known as Bourneville's disease after a French neurologist.

## Hair cycle

The phases of the hair's growth cycle are given by the acronym ACT.

**ACT**

| | |
|---|---|
| **Anagen** | (longest phase) |
| **Catagen** | |
| **Telogen** | (resting phase) |

Hair loss occurring about 3 months after pregnancy or major illness is considered as telogen-phase hair loss.

## Kaposi's sarcoma

KAPOSI reminds you what to look out for:

**KAPOSI**

| K | Conjunctivitis |
|---|---|
| A | AIDS-defining illness (1993 classification) |
| P | Palate lesions |
| O | Other sites (e.g. lungs and lymph nodes) |
| S | Skin |
| I | Indigestion (the GI tract is affected) |

# Papules

Papules are small and elevated skin lesions (unlike maculae). So remember:

**Papules are Palpable**

# Keratoacanthoma

Keratoacanthoma looks like a *volcano* because of a central keratin plug which often comes off. To remember this, remember the condition as:

**Krakatoa – Acanthoma!**

 **SWOT BOX**

Keratoacanthoma is an overgrowth of pilosebaceous glands (hair follicle cells) with potential for malignancy, although is self-limiting in most cases. It is often mistaken for a squamous cell carcinoma.

# Pemphigus vs pemphigoid

Is there an easy way to remember the difference between them? You bet!

| PemphiguS | Superficial |
|---|---|
| PemphigoiD | Deep |

 **SWOT BOX**

**Pemphigus** is a group of skin diseases with vesicles and bullae, acantholysis on histology and antiepidermal autoantibodies.

**Pemphigoid** has cleft formation at the dermoepidermal junction, while immunofluorescence reveals complement and IgG deposits at the level of the lamina lucida of the basement membrane. Yes, you've read it before.

# Ultraviolet A vs B

UVA rays penetrate through the epidermis better than UVB rays, so they have different effects in general.

| | |
|---|---|
| **UVA** | **Ageing (of the skin, wrinkles)** |
| **UVB** | **Burning, Browning and Blindness (cataracts)** |

# Xerostoma

Xerostoma means 'mouth dryness'. So think about this condition as *xerosaliva* – zero saliva.

**Zero saliva** makes your mouth dry!

# 7.5 ENDOCRINOLOGY

## Acromegaly

Amazingly, each of the first ten letters of the alphabet describes one or more features of acromegaly.

### A-B-C-D-E-F-G-H-I-J

| | |
|---|---|
| A | Arthropathy |
| B | Big boggy hands |
| C | Carpal tunnel syndrome |
| D | Diabetes |
| E | Enlarged tongue, heart and throat |
| F | Fields (bitemporal hemianopia) |
| G | Gynaecomastia, Galactorrhoea and Greasy skin |
| H | Hypertension (20–50%) |
| I | Increasing size (of shoes, hat, gloves, dentures, rings) |
| J | Jaw enlargement and prognathism |

## Carcinoid syndrome

Yet more amazingly, every letter of the word carcinoid describes one of its features.

### CARCINOID

| | |
|---|---|
| C | Cyanosis |
| A | Asthma |
| R | Rubor |
| C | Cor pulmonale |
| I | Incompetent tricuspid/pulmonary valve |
| N | Noisy abdomen |
| O | Oedema |
| I | Indoles in stools |
| D | Diarrhoea |

**SWOT BOX**

**Carcinoid tumours** are neuroendocrine in origin and produce a variety of different polypeptide hormones and products, especially serotonin (5-HT). Tumours are generally in the gastrointestinal tract and are often asymptomatic.

**Carcinoid syndrome** is usually associated with ileal carcinoids because hepatic decarboxylation is avoided.

# Cushing's

The important causes of Cushing's are easily remembered courtesy of Adrianne:

### Cushion Is Put On Top Of Adrienne's Stereo

| | |
|---|---|
| **Cush**ion is | **Cush**ing's |
| **Put on** | **P**ituitary adenoma |
| **Top** of | ec**TOP**ic ACTH |
| **Adr**ianne's | **Adr**enal tumour |
| **Ster**eo | **Ster**oids |

### *Alternative*

Adrianne's On Top – Put Stereo On!

# Diabetes mellitus

Complications of diabetes mellitus are indicated by KNIVES.

### KNIVES

| | | |
|---|---|---|
| **K** | **Kidney** | **Glomerular sclerosis; uraemia; hypertension; nephrotic syndrome; renal papillary necrosis; atherosclerosis of renal vessels; effects of hypertension** |

| N | Neuromuscular | Peripheral neuropathy; mononeuritis (see p. 108) autonomic neuropathy; diabetic amyotrophy |
|---|---|---|
| I | Infective | Urinary tract, skin and soft tissue infection; tuberculosis; moniliasis; pyelonephritis |
| V | Vascular | Large vessel → ischaemic heart disease<br>Small vessel → micrangiopathy |
| E | Eye | Cataracts; background proliferative and pre-proliferative retinopathy; microaneurysms; maculopathy; fibrosis; retinal detachment; photocoagulation spots of retinal burns |
| S | Skin | Lipoatrophy and insulin sensitivity at injection site; necrobiosis lipoidica; granuloma annulare |

# Diabetic ketoacidosis

I am grateful to Dr R Clarke of Barnet General Hospital for this suggested scheme pertaining to the emergency management of diabetic ketoacidosis (DKA).

### PANICS

| P | Potassium |
|---|---|
| A | Aspirate stomach (nasogastric tube) |
| N | Normal saline |
| I | Insulin infusion |
| C | Cultures (midstream urine, blood)/catheterize |
| S | Subcutaneous heparin |

# Anterior pituitary hormones

The six anterior pituitary hormones are thyroid-stimulating hormone (TSH), growth hormone (GH), the gonadotrophins (luteinizing hormone, LH, and follicle-stimulating hormone, FSH), prolactin and adrenocorticotrophic hormone (ACTH).

### Those Giant Gonads Prolong the Action

| | |
|---|---|
| **Those** | **TSH** |
| **Giant** | **GH** |
| **Gonads** | **LH/FSH** |
| **Prolong the** | **Prolactin** |
| **Action** | **ACTH** |

# Phaeochromocytoma

This is a usually benign, well-encapsulated lobular tumour of chromaffin cells in the adrenal medulla. It mainly presents as raised blood pressure (see CREEP on p. 82). Attacks also cause palpitations, sweating, tremor and nausea.

### 10 per cent rule

**10%** are multiple
**10%** are malignant
**10%** are adrenal bilateral
**10%** are extra-adrenal
**10%** are familial
**10%** are in children[3]

The 10% ACME rule has its place too:

### 10 per cent ACME

**10%** are:

| | |
|---|---|
| **A** | **Adrenal (bilateral)** |
| **C** | **Children** |
| **M** | **Malignant** |
| **E** | **Extra-adrenal** |

3 Figures from *Update* (10/6/1998) p. 1130.

# Parathyroid glands

There are four interesting facts about these glands.

## All 4s

**4 glands**
**4 th (and 3rd) branchial arch is where they arise from**
**40 mg in weight**
**40 mm in diameter**

# Secondary hyperparathyroidism

**Primary hyperparathyroidism** accounts for 30% of cases of raised calcium levels (remember: bones, stones, moans and abdominal groans). But in **secondary hyperparathyroidism** the calcium is lowered. This is because chronically low plasma calcium levels are the cause of the compensatory increase in PTH secretion. After reading Section III, try coming back to make a 'link' mnemonic for these 10 Cs.

## The 10 Cs of secondary hyperparathyroidism

**Calcium down**
**Cramps**
**Carpopedal spasms**
**Chvostek's sign**
**Convulsions**
**Cataracts**
**Cavities (dental)**
**Crazy (change in mental state)**
**Cardiac arrhythmias**
**Cranial pressure rises**

# Solitary thyroid nodules

To remember the causes, remember about the heroin, acid, hash and coke.

### Sold Students Heroin, Acid, Hash 'n' Coke

| | |
|---|---|
| **Sold** | **Sol**itary |
| **Students** | **C**ysts |
| **Heroin** | **H**aemorrhage |
| **Acid** | **A**denoma |
| **Hash** | **Hash**imoto's |
| **'n'** | big **N**odule |
| **Coke** | **C**arcinoma |

# Diffuse goitre

These are the causes.[4]

### Limp Simon's Silent Grave is Stashed with Hash

| | |
|---|---|
| **Limp** | **L**ymphoma |
| **Sim**on's | **Sim**ple non-toxic goitre |
| **Silent** | **Silent** thyroiditis (painless) |
| **Grave** is | **Grave**'s |
| **S**tashed with | **S**ubacute thyroiditis |
| **Hash** | **Hash**imoto's |

Here is another useful version.[5]

### Simple Substances Like Hash Get You Sex

| | |
|---|---|
| **Simple** | **Simple** non-toxic goitre |
| **Sub**stances | **Sub**acute thyroiditis |
| **L**ike | **L**ymphoma |
| **Hash** | **Hash**imoto's |
| **G**et you | **G**rave's |
| **S**ex | **S**ilent thyroiditis |

4  Contributed by Sana Haroon BSc (2007).
5  Contributed by Dr Majeed Mussalam BSc (2007).

# 7.6 GASTROENTEROLOGY

## Cirrhosis

The complications of cirrhosis are listed under PAPAH.

### PAPAH

| | |
|---|---|
| P | Portal hypertension |
| A | Ascites |
| P | Portosystemic encephalopathy |
| A | Acute renal failure |
| H | Hepatocellular carcinoma |

## Gastrointestinal bleeding

The causes of bleeding of the upper gastrointestinal tract are given by VARICES. There are idiopathic causes in 2–4% of cases.

| | |
|---|---|
| V | Varices |
| A | Alcohol and drugs |
| R | Rupture (Mallory–Weiss) |
| I | Idiopathic (in 2–4%) |
| C | Carcinoma |
| E | oEsophagitis or gastric Erosion |
| S | Stomach (gastric ulcer or duodenal ulcer) |

## Gum hypertrophy

A good way to remember the causes:

### Look! Funny Crowns!

| | |
|---|---|
| Look | Leukaemia |
| Funny | Phenytoin |
| Crowns | Crohn's or Ciclosporin |

# Hepatitis B

The risk groups for hepatitis B are given by the 6 Hs.[6]

### The 6 Hs of hepatitis B

**Health** workers (have you had your jabs yet?)
**Heroin** (or other intravenous drug abusers)
**Haemophiliacs**
**Homosexuals**
**Haemodialysis**
**Homes** (people in institutions)

# Hepatomegaly

Hepatomegaly has five main causes as described here.

### Hippies Sell Space In Congested Bedsit

| | |
|---|---|
| **Hip**pies | **Hep**atomegaly is caused by: |
| **Sell** | **Cell**ular proliferation |
| **Space** | **Space**-occupying lesions |
| **In** | **In**filtration |
| **Congested** | **Congest**ion |
| **BedSIT** | **Bil**E **D**uct ob**ST**ruction |

# Inflammatory bowel disease

Treatment of inflammatory bowel disease includes a number of drugs.

### Curt flogs Cyndi's Meaty Ass

| | |
|---|---|
| **Curt** | **C**orticosteroids |
| **Flogs** | **Fl**agyl (metronidazole) |
| **Cyndi's** | **C**iclosporins |
| **Meaty** | **M**ethotrexate |
| **Ass** | **A**zathioprine and **A**minosalicylates (5-ASA) |

6  Collier JAB, Longmore M, Brinsden M (1999) *Oxford Handbook of Clinical Specialties*, 5th edn. Oxford: Oxford University Press.

You may prefer this reminder:

### And as Curt Met Cindy

| And As | Azathioprine and Aminosalicylates (5-ASA) |
|--------|-------------------------------------------|
| Curt   | Corticosteroids                           |
| Met    | Methotrexate and Metronidazole            |
| Cindy  | Ciclosporins                              |

# Ulcerative colitis

The features of a severe attack of ulcerative colitis often involve low serum albumin (< 30 g/L), fever (> 37.5°C), anaemia (Hb < 10 g%), tachycardia, high erythrocyte sedimentation rate (ESR > 30 mm/hour) and bloody diarrhoea. A useful mnemonic is given here.

### SHITER

| S | Serum albumin ↓             |
|---|-----------------------------|
| H | High fever                  |
| I | Iron deficiency (anaemia)   |
| T | Tachycardia                 |
| E | ESR ↑                       |
| R | Red (blood) in diarrhoea    |

# Pancreatitis

Causes of pancreatitis are given by this very well-known mnemonic.

### GET SMASH'D

| G | Gallstones           |
|---|----------------------|
| E | Ethanol              |
| T | Trauma               |
| S | Steroids             |
| M | Mumps                |
| A | Autoimmune disease   |
| S | Scorpion bites       |
| H | Hyperlipidaemia      |
| D | Drugs                |

And the investigations of pancreatitis are encapsulated here:

## O, Claw Gut

| | |
|---|---|
| **O** | **O**xygen (blood gases) |
| **C** | **C**alcium |
| **L** | **L**actate dehydrogenase |
| **A** | **A**mylase |
| **W** | **W**hite cell count |
| **G** | **G**lucose |
| **U** | **U**rea |
| **T** | **T**ransaminase |

# 7.7 HAEMATOLOGY

## Direct Coombs test

This tests for haemolytic anaemia with an immune cause.

**HICCUP**

| | |
|---|---|
| **H** | **Haemolytic anaemia of…** |
| **I** | **Immunological…** |
| **C** | **Cause** $\rightarrow$ |
| **C** | **Coombs test is…** |
| **U** | **Usually…** |
| **P** | **Positive** |

## Anaemia

There are FIVE ways to treat anaemia.[7]

**FIVE**

| | |
|---|---|
| **F** | **Folate** |
| **I** | **Iron** |
| **V** | **Vitamin B12** |
| **E** | **Erythropoietin** |

## Favism (G6PD deficiency)

To remember that favism (G6PD deficiency) is associated with Heinz bodies in the red blood cell (on blood film or methyl violet stain) imagine a tin of Heinz 'Fava' Beans.

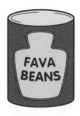

7 From Sarah Gates, St Andrews University, 2005.

**SWOT BOX**

The full name of the enzyme G6PD is **glucose-6-phosphate dehydrogenase**. It is involved in the **hexose monophosphate shunt** involved in glutathione reduction. It is essential for protecting red cell membranes from oxidative crises. If the cell is lacking in reduced glutathione, nothing protects the haemoglobin from being oxidized, precipitating rapid anaemia with jaundice.

The oxidized haemoglobin precipitates within the cell to form **Heinz bodies,** which stick to the membrane and make it more rigid.

**Splenic macrophages** lyse the inclusion-bearing cells. This can happen with fava beans (*Vicia faba*), illness, antimalarial drugs or other drugs such as sulphonamides.

# Haemophilias A and B

*Haemophilia A* is due to lack of factor 8 and *haemophilia B* is due to lack of factor 9. Think of:

Factor **8**      **A**ight (rather than Eight)
Factor **9**      **b** (upside down)

# Lymphadenopathy

Causes of lymph node enlargement include sarcoid, syphilis, metastatic disease (e.g. lympho- and reticulosarcomas), primary reticuloses, lymphogranuloma, glandular fever and TB.

### Sarcastic Sybil Met Trouble in Ridiculing Grannie's Gift

| | |
|---|---|
| **Sarcastic** | **Sarcoid** |
| **Sybil** | **Sy**philis |
| **Met** | **Met**astatic disease |
| **TrouBle** | **TuB**erculosis |
| **In** | **N**on-specific |
| **Ridiculing** | **R**eticuloses |
| **Grannie's** | lympho**GRAN**uloma |
| **GiFt** | **G**landular **F**ever |

# Sickle cell and glutamine

The sickle cell beta-globin gene causes valine to be replaced by glutamine at position 6. So think of:

### Glute's in position sex

| | |
|---|---|
| **Glut**e's in | **Glut**amine |
| Position **sex** | Position **six** |

Now, you already know that the homozygous state of the haemoglobin (Hb) structure in this condition is designated *HbSS*, and heterozygous as *HbAS*. So let us link *HbAS* to facts we need to learn:

### HbAS

| | |
|---|---|
| **H** | **Hypoxia, haemolytic crises** |
| **b** | **Beta chain affected** |
| **A** | **Aplastic crises, acute sequestration crises** |
| **S** | **Sixth position of Hb beta chain** |
| | **Symptoms start at age Six months (fetal Hb present before 6 months)** |
| | **Sodium metabisulphite test (induces Sickling *in vitro*)** |

# Unconjugated bilirubin

 **RAPID REVISION**

Here's a quick question for you. What are the causes of unconjugated bilirubin? If you don't know them yet, then check p. 66 for a cool mnemonic!

# 7.8 NEUROLOGY

*More brain, O Lord, more brain!*

George Meredith

## Gait abnormalities

The causes of abnormal gait are numerous, as summarized here.

### All Patients Spending Cash See Proper Doctors[8]

| | |
|---|---|
| **All** | **Apraxia/ataxia** |
| **Patients** | **Parkinsonism** |
| **Spending** | **Spasticity** |
| **Cash** | **Cerebellar ataxia** |
| **See** | **Sensory deficit** |
| **Proper** | **Proximal myopathy** |
| **Doctors** | **Distal myopathy** |

 **SWOT BOX**

**Apraxia** is the inability to perform learned voluntary movements in the absence of paralysis. If it involves the loss of writing ability, it is called **agraphia**.

## Epileptic seizures

This anonymous and ancient rhyme (from the days when the word 'fit' was widely used) neatly sums up the features of epileptic seizures.

**The aura, the cry, the fall, the fit**
**The tonus, the clonus, the piss and the shit**
**Describes an epileptic fit**

Obviously this describes the features of a *tonic* (spasm) and *clonic* (jerking) seizure. It is useful for determining whether or not the fit was epileptiform. You do, of course, need to be aware of the wide variety of clinical patterns of epilepsy – including altered motor and sensory phenomena, altered consciousness and sometimes odd behaviour.

See more on treatment of epilepsy on p. 53.

8 With thanks to Stuart McCorkel, SGMMS 1990.

# Cerebellar signs

This is a common subject in exams. It is definitely worth knowing the following mnemonic well.[9]

## DANISH

| | |
|---|---|
| **D** | **Dysdiadochokinesia** |
| **A** | **Ataxia** |
| **N** | **Nystagmus** |
| **I** | **Intention tremor (approx. 3 Hz)** |
| **S** | **Speech (Scanning/Staccato)** |
| **H** | **Hypotonia** |

 **SWOT BOX**

**Cerebellar signs** are ipsilateral to a lesion.

**Dysdiadochokinesia** is impairment in ability to perform rapidly alternating movements such as sequential supination and pronation.

**Ataxia** (Greek, *taxis* = order; *a* = negative) is lack of muscular coordination, and it leads to an abnormal gait; the patient often staggers and walks with a broad-based gait for stability, tending to fall in the direction of the side of the lesion.

**Cerebellar nystagmus** is usually horizontal (ask the patient to look laterally); the 'finger–nose' test shows the 'past-pointing' effect of the **intention tremor**, whereby on being asked to touch their nose, the patient misses and hits their cheek). Note that tremor is not affected by closing the eyes and occurs during a movement – not at rest (unlike Parkinson's disease).

**Speech** is often affected (dysarthria) and sometimes described as 'slurred and explosive'.

The **muscles** are often **hypotonic** but may be hypertonic also, which (of course) aggravates the ataxia.

---

9 From Dr Robert Clarke (2004–07) *Medicine for Finals*. Dr Clarke's Revision Courses in Association with the BMA.

# Claw hand

There are many causes of claw hand which this mnemonic may help you to remember.

### Um...VW Brake-Pads Made In Romania Suck

| | |
|---|---|
| **UM** | **U**lnar and **M**edian nerve palsy |
| **VW** | **V**olkmann's contracture (ischaemia) |
| **Brake-Pads** | **Brachial Plexus** lesion of... |
| **Made** | **M**edial cord |
| **In** | **In**jury |
| **Romania** | **R**heumatoid arthritis |
| **SuCk** | **S**pinal **C**ord lesion |

Among the injuries that cause claw hand are scarring, trauma and burns. The spinal cord lesions include polio, syringomyelia and lateral amyotrophic sclerosis (remember these as *Pull Strings Laterally, Amy*).

### Pull Strings Laterally, Amy

| | |
|---|---|
| **Pull** | **P**olio |
| **Strings** | **S**yringomelia |
| **Laterally** | **Lateral** |
| **Amy** | **Amy**otrophic sclerosis |

# Coma

You can distinguish between pontine and cerebral causes of coma by the direction of deviation of the eyes.

| | |
|---|---|
| **Pontine lesions** | Eyes **P**oint to **P**aralyzed limbs |
| **Cerebral lesion** | Eyes **S**tare at **S**atisfactory limbs |

 **SWOT BOX**

The eyes may deviate away from the midline due to cerebral hemisphere lesions where they 'look' towards the side of the lesion (i.e. towards the normal limbs). With pontine lesions this generally occurs in the opposite direction, so eyes deviate away from the side of the lesion towards the affected limbs.

# Examination

A simple mnemonic for remembering what to include in a standard neurological examination.[10]

### That Physician Really Is So Cool

| | |
|---|---|
| **That** | **Tone** |
| **Physician** | **Power** |
| **Really** | **Reflexes** |
| **Is** | **Inspection** |
| **So** | **Sensation** |
| **Cool** | **Coordination/orientation** |

# Friedreich's ataxia

These are the main features and associations.

### French Taxi Cars ARe Scarce, Babe

| | |
|---|---|
| **FRench** | **FRiedrich** |
| **TAXI** | **aTAXIa** |
| **CArs** | **CARdiomyopathy** |
| **ARe** | **Autosomal Recessive** |
| **SCarce** | **SColiosis** |
| **BABe** | **BABinski sign (positive: also have high arched plantars)** |

Note that the Babinski sign is present in patients with Friedrich's ataxia. They will also have high-arched plantars.

---

 **SWOT BOX**

**Friedrich's ataxia** is a hereditary spinocerebellar degenerative disease. It was named after Professor Nicholaus Friedreich, a German neurologist (1825–1882).

---

10 Attributed to Dr Sheetle Shah, Croydon.

# Gerstmann syndrome

This syndrome is a combination of four symptoms and can be remembered quite easily.

### A-ALF

| | |
|---|---|
| **A** | **Agraphia** |
| **A** | **Acalculia** |
| **L** | **Left–right disorientation** |
| **F** | **Finger agnosia** |

 **SWOT BOX**

**Gerstmann's** is due to a lesion in the angular gyrus of the dominant hemisphere. *Agraphia* means the inability to write. *Acalculia* is similar but relates to the ability to perform simple arithmetic calculations. *Agnosia* is the loss of recognition of sensory stimuli. The syndrome is named after Josef Gerstmann, a Viennese neurologist (1887–1969).

# Mononeuritis multiplex

SCALD will remind you of causes of this disease.

### SCALD

| | |
|---|---|
| **S** | **Sarcoid** |
| **C** | **Carcinoma** |
| **A** | **Arteritis** |
| **L** | **Leprosy** |
| **D** | **Diabetes** |

# Myotonic dystrophy

Popular in exams, this is a rare condition affecting only 5 in 10 000, which often becomes more severe in successive generations. Use the first nine letters of the alphabet to help you with some of the main features.

## A-B-C-D-E-F-G-H-I

**A**   Atrophy or if autosomal dominant

**B**   Baldness (frontal, in males)

**C**   Cataracts or if Chromosome 9 affected

**D**   Droopy eyes or Dysphagia or Diabetes (if end organs do not respond to insulin)

**E-F**   Expressionless Face or Forehead (from wasting of muscles of facial expression)

**G**   Gonadal atrophy (small pituitary fossa)

**H**   Heart (cardiomyopathy/conduction defects)

**I**   Immunology (low serum Ig) and Intellectual deterioration

---

 **SWOT BOX**

**Myotonia (droopy eyes)** is the inability of muscles to relax normally after contraction. It may be unilateral. In advanced disease it is less obvious, owing to muscle wasting. The resulting weakness is the main eventual cause of disability.

**Myotonic dystrophy** often manifests in adolescence or childhood and progresses thereafter. There is also an autosomal dominant congenital form (myotonia congenita) which can manifest itself *in utero*. To check for this, ask the patient to grip your fingers or shake your hand firmly, then let go as fast as possible. The delay in relaxation worsens in the cold and on excitation.

---

# Parkinson's disease

TRAP is a neat way to remember the clinical features of Parkinson's.

## TRAP

**T**   Tremor at rest (4–7 Hz)

**R**   Rigidity

**A**   Akinesia

**P**   Posture (simian) and gait (shuffling)

# Peripheral neuropathy

The five main causes conveniently start with the first five letters of the alphabet.[11]

## A-B-C-D-E

| | |
|---|---|
| A | Alcohol |
| B | B12 |
| C | Chronic renal failure and Carcinoma |
| D | Diabetes and Drugs |
| E | Every vasculitis |

# Reflexes

This is a popular and simple aide-memoir to remember which nerves relate to which reflexes.[12]

## AK-BeST

| | |
|---|---|
| A | Ankle (S1) |
| K | Knee (L2, L3, L4) |
| BeST | Biceps, Supinator (C5, C6) and Triceps (C7) |

 **SWOT BOX**

All the muscles on the dorsal aspect of the upper limb are innervated by C7 – in other words, the triceps, wrist and finger extensors.

# Restless legs syndrome

Considered to be a neurological sensorimotor disorder, this can be diagnosed using the URGE criteria.[13]

## URGE

| | |
|---|---|
| U | Urge – Is there an urge to move the legs? |
| R | Resting – Does resting bring it on? |
| G | Getting up – Does getting up and moving about help? |
| E | Evenings – Are evenings worse? |

11 From Dr Robert Clarke (2004–07) *Medicine for Finals.* Dr Clarke's Revision Courses in Association with the BMA.
12 Faisal Raza, University of East Anglia.
13 Allen RP, Picchietti D, Hening WA, Trenkwalder C, Walters AS, Montplaisir J (2003) Restless legs syndrome: diagnostic criteria, special considerations, and epidemiology. *Sleep Medicine* **4**:101–19.

# 7.9 RENAL MEDICINE AND UROLOGY

## Cystinuria

In this hereditary condition, four dibasic amino acids are not reabsorbed by the proximal convoluted tubule (i.e. cystine, ornithine, arginine and lysine). Use COAL to remind you of these:

**COAL**

| | |
|---|---|
| **C** | **Cystine** |
| **O** | **Ornithine** |
| **A** | **Arginine** |
| **L** | **Lysine** |

 **SWOT BOX**

The main consequence is that cystine stones are formed in the renal tract (cystine is the least soluble so it forms the stones). Note that cystine stones are seen on X-ray (but are less radiopaque than calcium stones).

## DMSA and DTPA

Two important radiological investigations of renal integrity are the DMSA and DTPA scans:

- [$^{99m}$Tc]DMSA is bound to proximal convoluted tubules in the cortex but gives little indication of the physiological function (e.g. urine production).
- *[$^{99m}$Tc]DTPA is given intravenously; a renogram curve shows vascular, secretory and excretory phases.

Highly technical so far, but this helps:

| | |
|---|---|
| **DTPA** | **Does The Physiology** |
| **DMSA** | **Doesn't Move** |

# Prostatic hypertrophy

A quarter to half of all men in their 40s and 50s have benign prostate hypertrophy.[14]

[Think of 1/4 to 50% in age 40–50]
60% of men in their **sixties**
70% of men in their **seventies**
80% of men in their **eighties**

# Causes of single solid scrotal mass

GHOST

| | |
|---|---|
| G | Gumma (nodile in tertiary stage syphilis) |
| H | Haematocele |
| O | Orchitis |
| S | Small testes with large epididymis found in epidiymitis |
| T | Tumour and Torsion |

# Causes of urethral stricture

Congenital (e.g. pinhole meatus)
Urethral valves
Neoplastic
Trauma (e.g. surgery, injury, foreign body)
*and*
Inflammation (gonorrhoea, meatal ulceration)

You can use the anagram **TUNIC**, or a suitable equivalent.

---

14  Data from Forte, Vincent, 'Ten Tips of Treating Enlarged Prostate', *Doctor newspaper*, June 2000.

# Chapter Eight

# PAEDIATRICS

## Apgar score

Here's a mnemonic used in daily clinical practice all over the world – a great one to show those who tell you they've never used mnemonics!

**APGAR** stands for **A**ppearance (colour of trunk), **P**ulse, **G**asp (respiratory effort), **A**ctivity (muscle tone), and **R**esponse to stimulation (e.g. irritating the sole).

| APGAR SCORE | 0 | 1 | 2 |
|---|---|---|---|
| Appearance | Pink | Blue limbs | All over blue |
| Pulse | 0 | <100 | >100 |
| Gasp | Absent | Irregular | Regular/crying |
| Activity | Flaccid | Diminished; limb flexion | Active movement |
| Response to stimulation | None | Poor (e.g. grimace) | Good (e.g. crying) |

## SWOT BOX

Virginia Apgar (1909–1974) was an American anaesthetist whose proposal for this scoring system was published in 1953. In 1963 the acronym APGAR was devised and coauthored with Dr J. Butterfield in the *Journal of the American Medical Association* and since has become one of the most utilized mnemonics in medicine.

The score is usually taken at 1 minute and at 5 minutes after delivery.

A score of < 4 in the first minute indicates that intubation should be considered (especially if score is falling).

Babies with this score have a 17% mortality rate (48% if have low birth weight), and with a score of < 4 at 5 minutes there is a 44% mortality.

# Blood pressure

A quick formula for BP *in kids* is:

$$\frac{90 + \text{age (in years)}}{55 + \text{age (in years)}}$$

# Body weight

A child's approximate weight is given by:

$$(\text{age in years} + 4) \times 2$$

For infants:

| Weight | Age (months) |
|--------|--------------|
| 6 kg   | 3/12         |
| 8 kg   | 6/12         |
| 9 kg   | 9/12         |
| 10 kg  | 12/12        |

# Breathing (respiratory) rates

Here they are, by age:

| Age | Approximate respirations/min |
|-----|------------------------------|
| 1 month | 60 |
| 1 year | 30 |
| 10 years | 15 |

# Breast feeding

Look at all these advantages of BREASTMILK!

**BREASTMILK**

| | |
|---|---|
| **B** | Bonding |
| **R** | Reduced solute |
| **E** | Eczema |
| **A** | Allergy protection |
| **S** | Sterilization not required |
| **T** | Taurine |
| **M** | Macrophages |
| **I** | Immunoglobulin A; higher IQ |
| **L** | Lactoperoxidase, Lysosymes, Lactoferrrin and Long chain fatty acids |
| **K** | Cot death (lower incidence) |

Remember, too, that:

**Cows' milk Contains Casein – Curd protein**

And that:

**Human milk Has more wHey**

**SWOT BOX**

A milk formula will resemble human milk more closely if it has a high **whey** to **curd** ratio. Higher-curd formulas are marketed 'for hungrier babies'.

*Note:* 1 oz equals 30 mL.

Breast fed babies are protected from **allergies** and are less likely to be intolerant to cow's-milk protein. Studies show they have a lower incidence of **eczema** and a higher **IQ** due to long chain fatty acids in the breastmilk. **Long chain fatty acids** are added to some formulas. Breastmilk also contains **macrophages** that kill bacteria, **lysosymes**, **lactoferrrin** which promotes **lactobacilli** and inhibits *Escherichia coli*, and **taurine** which aids development. It also has reduced levels of **solutes** like sodium, phosphate and proteins compared with formula milk.

# Chromosome disorders

Three **trisomies** and their affected chromosomes:

**PED**

| P | Patau's (+18) |
| E | Edward's (+13) |
| D | Down's (+21) |

Four **chromosome deletions** to remember:

**Delete That Horny Wolf I Prayed You Will Chat With An Angel**

| **Delete** That | Deletions |
| **Horny Wolf** | **Wolf**–Hirsch**horn** syndrome (4p-) |
| **Prayed** You **Will** | **Prader Willi** (chromosome 15) |
| **Chat** | Cri du **chat** (5p-) |
| **Angel** | **Angleman's** (chromosome 15) |

# Cytomegalovirus

Here are 3 important facts about CMV.

### The three 3s

**3% is the rate of primary infection (this is the commonest primary infection in pregnancy)**

**30% is the risk of transmission to the fetus (half are due to reactivation of the virus)**

**3 per 1000 births is the UK incidence**

 **SWOT BOX**

95% of affected infants with **cytomegalovirus infection** are asymptomatic, although 10% of these may become deaf in later life. There is 30% mortality rate for those with severe congenital disease.

**Complications** include low birth weight, neurological sequelae, abortion, anaemia, hydrops, pneumonitis and purpura. **Investigations** include CMV on throat swab, urine, infant serum Ig M. Transfusion services provide CMV-screened blood for neonates.

# Developmental dysplasia of the hip

Developmental dysplasia of the hip (DDH) is associated with these risk factors:

### The 7 Fs of DDH

**Fetal factors (such as multiple pregnancies)**
**Floppy (hypotonia)**
**Feet first (more common in breech presentation)**
**First born**
**Female**
**Family history**
**Freezing (said to be more common in winter-born babies)**

While the gold-standard screening test for dysplastic or dislocated hips in infants is the ultrasound, in UK practice most babies are not screened this way and we still rely on visual checks of symmetry of creases and Barlow's and Ortolani's tests. These test can only be done up to about 3 months of age (too much muscle tone in limbs beyond this age makes the tests very painful).

**Barlow's test** is for a *dislocataBle* hip. The hip is flexed to 90 degrees and adducted. Then the femoral head is pushed posteriorly, while internally rotating. A dislocatable hip will 'clunk' as it slips over the rim of the acetabulum.

**Ortolani's** test is for a hip that is *already* dislocated. This can be done next. The hips and knees are flexed with your middle finger over the greater trochanter and your thumb along the medial femur. Pull the hip gently forwards while abducting.

To summarize:

**Barlow's is Backwards**
**Ortolani's is Outwards**

# Fallot's tetralogy

Fallot's trilogy is **R**ight ventricular hypertrophy, **A**SD and **P**ulmonary stenosis – **RAP**. Then there's this:

### Fella's Blue – Pull His *Vesd* Right Over

| | |
|---|---|
| **Fella's** | **Fallot**'s |
| **Blue** | **C**yanotic |
| **Pull** his | **Pul**monary stenosis |
| **VeSD** | **VSD** (ventricular septal defect) |
| **Right** | **Right** ventricular hypertrophy |
| **Over** | **Over**-riding aorta |

 **SWOT BOX**

Etienne-Louis Arthur Fallott (1850–1911) was Professor of Hygiene and Legal Medicine at Marseilles. However, **Fallot's tetralogy** was first described by the Danish anatomist, geologist, Catholic priest and physician Niels Stensen (1638–1686) to an Italian court. He also named the female gonad as the *ovary* (which was previously thought of as a female testis) and postulated that it was analogous to the egg-laying organ of birds.

# Febrile convulsions

The Febrile 5s are useful here.

### Febrile 5s
**5 months to 5 years is approx. age range affected**
**5% of children affected**
**50% recurrence rate**

# Gum hypertrophy

 **RAPID REVISION**

You may remember the causes of gym hypertrophy from 'Look! Funny Crowns'. They are leukaemia, phenytoin and Crohn's or ciclosporin.

# Innocent murmur

You should know the 'S' signs of an innocent murmur:

### The 6 S signs
**Symptom free**
**Systolic**
**Split-second sound**
**Sternal edge (left) side**
**Small part of pulmonary area only**
**Signs are otherwise normal**

# Kawasaki disease

This is also known as mucocutaneous lymph node syndrome. The CRESTS signs apply here:

## CRESTS

C     Cervical lymphadenopathy; C-reactive protein raised

R     Rash (widespread, polymorphic)

E     Eyes (bilateral, non-exudative conjunctivitis)

S     Strawberry tongue; red lips

T     Temperature raised (persists over 5 days, unresponsive to antibiotics and antipyretics)

S     Sausage-like fingers/toes from oedema
      Skin on palms/soles peeling

# Mumps – still moping??

 **SWOT BOX**

**Mumps** is caused by an airborne **paramyxovirus** (it is also spread by direct contact via body fluids). Uncommon in adults, it is often subclinical in children. Salivary gland inflammation is often the principal manifestation (e.g. parotitis, either uni- or bilateral).

**Complications** include epididymo-orchitis, oophoritis, meningoencephalitis and pancreatitis. Mumps meningitis is usually benign (vomiting, neck rigidity, lethargy, headache, photophobia, convulsions, abdominal pain and fever).

Investigations include cerebrospinal fluid (CSF), positive throat swab, stool culture and rising titre on serum antibody.

*This MOPE mnemonic was explained on p. 59. It stands for meningism, orchitis/oophoritis, parotitis/pancreatitis/paramyxovirus and encephalitis.*

# Nappy rash

Some of the causes are given here.

**PEE-SAC**

| | |
|---|---|
| **P** | **Psoriasis** |
| **E** | **Eczema** |
| **E** | **Excoriation (e.g. due to diarrhoea, acid stools, disaccharide intolerance, etc.)** |
| **S** | **Seborrhoeic dermatitis** |
| **A** | **Ammoniacal dermatitis** |
| **C** | **Candidiasis** |

# Recessive genetic disorders

A helpful rhyme about some autosomal recessive conditions:

A sick taxi driver named **Fred**
A **Thali** he'd had before bed
Dr **Hoffman** was called
But his **girdle** was mauled
So **incysted** I **PicK U** instead!

And this is what it all means:

| | |
|---|---|
| **Fred** | **Fried**rich's Ataxia (see section TK) |
| **Thali** | **Thal**assemia |
| **Hoffman** | Werdnig–**Hoffman** |
| **Girdle** | Limb **girdle** dystrophy |
| **Incysted** | **Cyst**ic fibrosis |
| **PicKU** | **PKU** (phenylketonuria) |

Here are some **X-linked recessive disorders**:

### Bright Rats with VD Are Incontinent

| | |
|---|---|
| **Bright** | Al**bright** syndrome |
| **Rats with** | **Rett** syndrome |
| **VD** a**Re** | Vitamin **D-R**esistant rickets |
| **Incontinent** | **Incontinent**ia pigmenti |

# TORCH'S infections

These are important non-bacterial infections that can affect the fetus:

## TORCH'S

| | |
|---|---|
| **T** | **Toxoplasmosis (see below)** |
| **O** | **Other STDs (e.g. syphilis)** |
| **R** | **Rubella (an RNA virus)** |
| **C** | **Cytomegalovirus (see below)** |
| **H** | **Herpes (e.g. chickenpox)** |
| **S** | **Slapped cheek (parvovirus B19)** |

# Toxoplasmosis

This 'tOXO' tetrad is shown here.

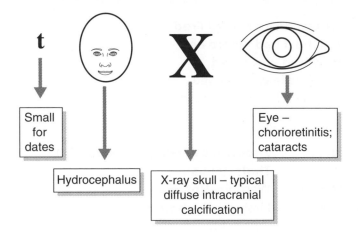

Small for dates

Hydrocephalus

X-ray skull – typical diffuse intracranial calcification

Eye – chorioretinitis; cataracts

**SWOT BOX**

The protozoan *Toxoplasma gondii* has its sexual cycle in the cat. It enters the human food chain by ingestion of oocytes (obtained via raw meat from other animals). Around 75% of the UK population are susceptible to this, however the vertical transmission rate is only 1 in 100 and only 10% of affected fetuses are damaged. Infected patients may be totally asymptomatic or may develop a non-specific illness with fatigue and flu-like symptoms.

Twelve cases are reported annually to the CDSU (Communicable Diseases Surveillance Unit). Pregnant women found to have seroconverted may be treated with three-weekly courses of spiramycin to reduce risk to the fetus. Infected neonates may be treated with spiramycin alternating with pyrimethamine + sulfadiazine.

# Chapter Nine

# SURGERY

*This chapter covers general surgery and surgery within the disciplines of orthopaedics, ENT and ophthalmology.*

## ? PRE-QUIZ

1 Can you describe the branches of the renal artery?
2 What should you ask in the history of a person with jaundice?
3 Who traditionally are said to get gallstones?
4 Do you remember which eye muscles are innervated by the IIIrd cranial nerve?
5 What are the signs of an arterial thrombus?
6 Can you name the ocular sign of syphilis?
7 What features on a mole imply a high suspicion of malignancy?
8 Which non-absorbable sutures can you name?

# 9.1 GENERAL SURGERY

## A surgical sieve

VITAMIN C DIP is a sieve for aetiologies of various pathologies. It's completely daft but it works something like this:

### VITAMIN C DIP

| | |
|---|---|
| V | Vascular |
| I | Infective |
| T | Trauma |
| A | Allergy/immunological |
| M | Metabolic/endocrine |
| I | Iatrogenic |
| N | Neoplastic |
| C | Congenital |
| D | Degenerative |
| i | Idiopathic |
| P | Psychogenic |

Here are two more old favourites:

### In A Surgeon's Gown, Physicians Might Make Some Progress

| | |
|---|---|
| **In** | Incidence |
| **A** | Age |
| **Surgeon's** | Sex |
| **Gown** | Geography |
| **Physicians** | Predisposing factors |
| **Might** | Macroscopic |
| **Make** | Microscopic |
| **Some** | Surgery |
| **Prog**ress | **Prog**nosis |

In A Surgeon's Gown, A Physician Can Cause
Inevitable Damage To Patients

| | |
|---|---|
| **In** | Incidence |
| **A** | Age |
| **Surgeon's** | Sex |
| **Gown** | Geography |
| **A** | Aetiology |
| **Physician** | Pathology |
| **Can** | Clinical presentation |
| **Cause** | Complications |
| **Inevitable** | Investigations |
| **Damage** | Differential diagnosis |
| **To** | Treatment |
| **Patients** | Prognosis |

# Intestinal obstruction

Remember the symptoms like this.

**Vomit PAD**

| | |
|---|---|
| **Vomit** | **Vomit**ing |
| **P** | **P**ain |
| **A** | **A**bsolute constipation |
| **D** | **D**istended |

# Abdominal distension (causes)

**The 6 Fs**

A **F**latulent **F**at **F**etus **F**loats in **F**luid **F**aeces

# Arterial thrombus

### The P signs

**Pale/pallor**

**Painful**

**Pulseless**

**Paralyzed**

**Paraesthesia**

**Perishing with cold!**

# Battle's sign

This is bruising behind the ear from a posterior fossa fracture. It is a sign of major trauma. W.H. Battle (1855–1936) was a surgeon at St Thomas's. Use simple pattern recognition here:

**Imagine being hit on the back of the head in a battle**

# Breast cancer

### D's nipple changes[1]

**Deviation**

**Depression**

**Destruction**

**Displacement**

**Deviation**

**Discharge**

**Duplication**

---

1 Modified from Browse N, Black J, Burnand KG, Thomas WEG (2005) *Browse's Introduction to Symptoms and Signs of Surgical Disease*, 4th edn. London: Arnold.

# Burns[2]

### The rule of 9s

| | |
|---|---|
| Back of trunk | $9\% \times 2$ |
| Front of trunk | $9\% \times 2$ |
| Each arm | 9% |
| Each leg | 9% |
| Head and neck | 9% |
| Perineum | 1% |
| Hand | 1% |

*Note:* Do not include simple erythema in the estimate.

# Central abdominal pain

If it's **acute** here are some possible causes:

### Your Terrible Ties Make Gas in Uranus

| | |
|---|---|
| **Your** | **Yersinia** |
| **Terrible** | **Tuberculosis** |
| **Ties** | **Typhoid** |
| **Make** | **Meckel's** |
| **Gas** | **Gastroenteritis** |
| **IN** | **INflammatory bowel disease (IBD)** |
| **URanus** | **URinary tract infection** |

And if it's **chronic** the causes may include:

### Sticking Radios in Cranes Can End the Burglaries

| | |
|---|---|
| **Sticking** | **Adhesions** |
| **Radios** | **Radiation** |
| **In** | **Ischaemia of bowel** |
| **Cranes** | **Crohn's** |
| **Can** | **Cancer** |
| **End** | **Endometriosis** |
| **The Burglaries** | **TB** |

2  From Collier JAB, Longmore M, Brinsden M (1999) *Oxford Handbook of Clinical Specialties*, 5th edn. Oxford: Oxford University Press.

# Clover leaf haemorrhoids

These are analogous to a **clover leaf** at positions 3 o'clock, 7 o'clock and 11 o'clock. External haemorrhoids are varicosities of the inferior rectal vein tributaries.

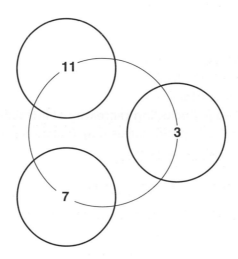

# Dukes cancer staging

Dukes staging for colon cancer (modified) goes like this:

| DUKES **A** | **A**-OK (best prognosis) – in bowel wall only |
| DUKES **B** | **B**reached Bowel wall |
| DUKES **C** | **C**olonic regional nodes |
| DUKES **D** | **D**istant metastases |

# Gallstones

Another anonymous aide memoire for the risk factors for gallstones.

**The 5 Fs**

**Fair**
**Fat**
**Female**
**Forty**
**Fertile**

# Jaundice

When taking a history from somebody with jaundice you may find the mnemonic CATHODES helpful.

## CATHODES

| | |
|---|---|
| C | Contacts |
| A | Anaemia |
| T | Travel |
| H | Had it before |
| O | Operations |
| D | Drugs (including recreational intravenous use) |
| E | Extra-hepatic causes (e.g. gallstones, sickle cell) |
| S | Sexual preference |

# Management of cases

If you're ever in an OSCE or viva and you get stuck on a question of how to manage a case, a useful tip is TIE (backwards!):

| | |
|---|---|
| E | Explanation to the patient |
| I | Investigation |
| T | Treatment |

*While there is tea, there is hope*
Sir Arthur Pinero (1855–1934)

# Meckel's diverticulum

This is part of the vitello-intestinal duct which completely disappears in 98% of the population. It causes complications such as perforation, and haemorrhage from peptic ulceration, obstruction (as it contains cells similar to those from stomach or pancreas).

A Meckel's diverticulum follows this rule of 2s.

## Rule of 2s

**2% of the population affected**
**2 to 1 male to female ratio**
**2 inches long**
**2 feet from the iliocaecal valve (on the antimesenteric border of the small intestine)**

**SWOT BOX**

J.F. Meckel the Younger (1781–1833) studied medicine at Vienna and discovered the first branchial cartilage. His grandfather first described the sphenopalatine ganglion, and his father was a Professor of Anatomy and Surgery.

# Melanoma

ABCD–BITCHES helps us here. How?

### A-B-C-D–BITCHES

| | |
|---|---|
| **A** | **Asymmetry (irregular)** |
| **B** | **Border (notched, indistinct or ulcerated)** |
| **C** | **Colour (increasingly variegated, especially black/grey)** |
| **D** | **Depth (of invasion)** |
| **B** | **Bleeding** |
| **I** | **Itching (persistent)** |
| **T** | **Tethering** |
| **C** | **Colour** |
| **H** | **Halo** |
| **E** | **Eczema-like features** |
| **S** | **Size (rapidly increasing) and Satellites (presence of)** |

# Pain characteristics

Bear in mind LOST WARD as you ask about the characteristics of pain.

### LOST WARD

| | |
|---|---|
| **L** | **Location** |
| **O** | **Onset/duration** |
| **S** | **Severity** |
| **T** | **Transmission/radiation** |
| **W** | **What...** |
| **A** | **Aggravates or...** |
| **R** | **Relieves** |
| **D** | **Duration/previous diagnoses** |

Alternatively, try the SOCRATES approach:

## SOCRATES

| | |
|---|---|
| **S** | **Site** |
| **O** | **Onset/duration** |
| **C** | **Character** |
| **R** | **Transmission/radiation** |
| **A** | **Aggravates or relieves?** |
| **T** | **Timing** |
| **E** | **Earlier diagnosis** |
| **S** | **Severity** |

# Raynaud's phenomenon

Raynaud's disease is most common in young women (60–90% of reported cases) and is idiopathic, hence:

**Raynaud's Disease we Don't know**
**Phenomenon has a Pathological cause**

Some of the causes are listed here, made more memorable by this naughty mnemonic.

## My Servant's Vibrator's So Cold, Ergo Dames Thighs Are Nervous

| | |
|---|---|
| **My** | **Malnutrition** |
| **Servant's** | **Cervical rib** |
| **Vibrator** | **Vibrat**ing tools |
| **So** | **Subclavian aneurysm and Stenosis (cause emboli)** |
| **Cold** | **Cold** exposure and **Col**lagen diseases |
| **Ergo** | **Ergo**t |
| **DaMes** | **Diabetes Mellitus** |
| **Thighs** | **Thy**roid deficiency |
| **Are** | **Atherosclerosis/Buerger's disease** |
| **Nerv**ous | **Neur**ological causes (e.g. spinal cord disease) |

*Note:* Also **WBC** gives **W**hite, **B**lue and **C**rimson, the order of the sequential colour changes of the hand seen in Raynaud's phenomenon.

**SWOT BOX**

Raynaud's phenomenon is secondary to other conditions, such as connective tissue disorders (scleroderma, rheumatoid arthritis, systemic lupus erythematosus), obstructive arterial diseases (e.g. thoracic outlet syndrome), neurogenic lesions, drug intoxications (ergot, methysergide), dysproteineamias and myxoedema.

# Sprain treatment

A very common mnemonic in clinical practice used by many health professionals.

## RICE

| | |
|---|---|
| **R** | **Rest** |
| **I** | **Ice (cold pack, e.g. frozen peas, or gel pack)** |
| **C** | **Compression (tubular crepe bandage)** |
| **E** | **Elevation (keep affected limb elevated)** |

If using ice crush it, wrap it up in layers of towelling and apply for 10–15 minutes, but not directly to the skin. If using peas, do not eat them! Mark the bag with a big 'X' to avoid possible food poisoning.

# Sutures

Here are some common types and brand names of **non-absorbable** sutures:

## SLEEP

| | |
|---|---|
| **S** | **Silk** |
| **L** | **Linen** |
| **E** | **Ethilon™** |
| **E** | **Ethibond™** |
| **P** | **Prolene™** |

And some **absorbable** ones:

## VCD

| | |
|---|---|
| **V** | **Vicryl™ (70 days)** |
| **C** | **Catgut** |
| **D** | **Dexon™** |

# 9.2 ORTHOPAEDICS

## Charcot's joints

Causes of Charcot's joints to remember.

### Charred lepers could syringe deaf tabby

| | |
|---|---|
| **Charred** | **Charcot's** |
| **Lepers** | **Leprosy** |
| **Could** | **Cauda** equine lesion |
| **Syringe** | **Syringomyelia (cyst in spinal cord)** |
| **Deaf** | **Diabetes** |
| **Tabby** | **Tabes dorsalis (degenerative condition of neurons)** |

 **SWOT BOX**

J.M. Charcot (1825–1893) was a famous French neurologist who introduced the study of geriatrics. He also studied hypnosis and art.

## Developmental dysplasia of the hip

Developmental dysplasia of the hip (DDH) is associated with the 7Fs as described on p. 117, where you will find much more on the subject. Previously this was described as congenital dislocation of the hip.

### All Fs

**Fetal factors (such as multiple pregnancies)**
**First born**
**Female**
**Family History**
**Floppy (hypotonia)**
**Feet first (more common in breech presentation)**

# Hammer or mallet toe

Hammer is a *proximal* flexion deformity, but mallet is a *distal* deformity.

**Hammer (proximal) then Mallet (distal) in alphabetical order!**

# Kyphosis or scoliosis

*Kyphosis* is anterior curvature of the spine and *scoliosis* is lateral curvature of the spine. This picture will help you remember.

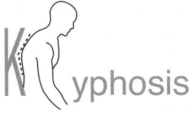

Kyphosis anterior curvature of the spine

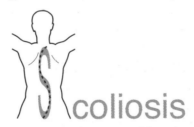

Scoliosis lateral curvature of the spine

Causes of this **kyphosis** are given by:

**Uncle Spikes Tabby Met Oscar's Kangaroo**

| | |
|---|---|
| **Uncle** | **Anky**losing |
| **Spikes** | **Spondylitis** |
| **TaBby** | **TB** |
| **Met** | **Met**astatic carcinoma |
| **Oscar's** | **Osteoporosis** |
| **Kangaroo** | **Congenital** |

# Valgum and varum

Genu *valgum* is *knock*-knees and genu *varum* is bow knees. Can you remember that?

**Valgum**      Imagine a *genie* who *knocks* his knees together modestly so he doesn't appear *vulgar*!

**Varum**       When they are bowed, the knees are *far from* each other (rhymes with *varum*)

# 9.3 EAR, NOSE AND THROAT

## Cholesteatomas

It's easy to remember that cholesteatomas often lead to *attic* perforations:

**Coal in the attic**

 **SWOT BOX**

This is a mass of keratinizing stratified squamous epithelium from the middle ear or mastoid cavity which can enlarge and damage or erode local tissue. It may be due to negative middle-ear pressure which then retracts the tympanic membrane – usually in the **attic** region.

## Deafness

When testing for **nerve deafness**, remember:

**Norm's Nerve PoWeR!**

| | |
|---|---|
| **Norm's** | **Norm**al ear in... |
| **Nerve** | **Nerve** deafness |
| **PoWeR** | **P**ositive **We**ber's and **R**inne's |

When testing for **conductive deafness**, remember:

**CD–WP**

| | |
|---|---|
| **C** | **C**onductive |
| **D** | **D**eafness is... |
| **W** | **W**eber's |
| **P** | **P**ositive |

## Rinne's and Weber's tests

In **Rinne's test** a tuning fork is applied to the mastoid, then it is placed near the ear, without any contact (held in the air). Rinne's test is a test of air conduction vs mastoid bone conduction. A 'positive' Rinne's means the note is heard *louder* in the *normal* ear. In Rinne's Rs are +ve.

## If Air Near Ear Is Louder It Is Normal

| | |
|---|---|
| ai**R** | **R** |
| nea**R** | **R** |
| ea**R** | **R** |
| loude**R** | **R** |
| no**R**mal | **R** |

In **Weber's test** the tuning fork is placed once on the midline of the head (e.g. top of the head or forehead). The letter '**W**' has a *midline*. You will now know (permanently) that Weber's is the test which involves touching the tuning fork on the *middle* of the head! So for Weber's test, remember:

## W for middle

**Weber's**        **W** *midline* means *middle*

*Note:* In these test 'positive' usually means 'louder'.

# 9.4 OPHTHALMOLOGY

## Fundoscopy

Where should you look on fundoscopy?

**DM–FT**

| | |
|---|---|
| **DM** | **Disc is Medial** |
| **FT** | **Fovea is Temporal** |

## Optic nerve (cranial II)

If asked to examine the function of the optic nerve, one possible scheme is AFRO:[3]

**AFRO**

| | |
|---|---|
| **A** | **Acuity** |
| **F** | **Fields** |
| **R** | **Reflexes (light/accommodation)** |
| **O** | **Optic disc** |

*Note:* Do the optic discs *last* of all – using the bright light constricts the pupil. PERLA is an acronym for Pupils Equal and Reactive to Light and Accommodation.

Having examined the optic disc (or 'papilla') you may see it is choking in fluid (choked disc = papilloedema). You will know this from the features CCCP.

## Papilloedema

The main features of the **choked disc** are given by CCCP.

**CCCP**

| | |
|---|---|
| **C** | **Colour change...** |
| **C** | **Contour and...** |
| **C** | **Cupping imply...** |
| **P** | **Papilloedema** |

---

3 With acknowledgement to Dr Lisa Culliford of St Georges' Hospital Medical School.

# Chapter Ten

# OBSTETRICS AND GYNAECOLOGY

## Antepartum haemorrhage

The causes of APH can be remembered using the acronym APH!

**APH**

| | |
|---|---|
| **A** | **Abruption** |
| **P** | **Placenta praevia (or vasa praevia)** |
| **H** | **Hardly known (40% are idiopathic)** |

## Cytomegalovirus

Remember the **3** CMV-related facts described on p. 117.[1] To recap:

### The 3s of cytomegalovirus
**3% is the rate of primary infection**
**30% risk of transmission to fetus**
**3 per 1000 births, UK incidence**

You'll find more information in the chapter on Paediatrics.

---

1 Figures from Gilbertson NJ, Walker S (1993) *Notes for the DCH*, 1st edn. Edinburgh: Churchill Livingston.

# Forceps delivery

A few things to remember when forceps delivery is likely.

### FORCEPS

| | |
|---|---|
| **F** | **Fully dilated** |
| **O** | **Occiput presentation** |
| **R** | **Ruptured membranes** |
| **C** | **Catheter to empty bladder** |
| **E** | **Engaged** |
| **P** | **Pain relief should be adequate** |
| **S** | **Space/Scissors (episiotomy)** |

But can you remember which forceps to use for high, low and middle cavities? Try this:

### WAK

| | | |
|---|---|---|
| **W** | **Wrigley's** | **Low** |
| **A** | **Anderson's** | **Mid** |
| **K** | **Kielland's (rotational)** | **High** |

*Note:* the use of Ventouse has largely superseded the high-cavity forceps.

# Meig syndrome

Meig syndrome is an ovarian tumour associated with ascites and pleural effusion or hydrothorax. J. V. Meigs was a Professor of Gynaecology at Harvard. Now think of a HAT for its main features.

### HAT

| | |
|---|---|
| **H** | **Hydrothorax** |
| **A** | **Ascites** |
| **T** | **Tumour of ovary** |

## *Alternative*

**PAT where P is for Pleural effusion.**

# Pelvic dimensions

The following 11–12–13 rule helps you with the (approximate) ideal female pelvic dimensions. These are approximate anterior–posterior (AP) dimensions.

## Pelvic Dimensions 11–12–13

**11 cm (AP) × 13 cm (transversely)**
**12 cm (mid-cavity of pelvis)**
**13 cm (AP) × 11 cm (transversely)**

The pelvic inlet is wider transversely and the outlet is wider anteroposteriorly.

The variation in diameter through the pelvis is a human characteristic – an adaptation to bipedal stance – which helps one walk upright but makes the second stage of labour more difficult for the fetus whose head must rotate to negotiate the variable shape of the pelvic 'tunnel'.

# Sperm counts – the norms

Here's a guide to the Norms (anonymous again, and apologies to Norm). Think of this as a sequence 2–2–4–6 in which the sperm count may be considered to have the following normal values:

## 2–2–4–6

**20 million is the minimum count in...**
**2 mL of which at least...**
**40% are motile and at least...**
**60% have normal morphology**

# Sterilization counselling

These are the issues involved in counselling before FEMALE sterilization.

## FEMALE

**F**     **Failure rate (1 in 500)**

**E**     **Ectopics (small relative increase in risk)**

**M**    **Menstrual changes (not taking the 'pill' any more)**

**A**     **Ain't reversible**

**L**     **Laparoscopic procedure (may be done at Caesarean section if baby is healthy)**

**E**     **Enter in notes ('Informed of failure rate and knows irreversible')**

See Chapter 8 Paediatrics for more information on events that can affect the fetus.

# Chapter Eleven

# PSYCHIATRY

## Delusional disorders

**Classification** of these is simple.

### Persistent Flies in Pairs Make Me Paranoid

| | |
|---|---|
| **Persistent** | **Persistent** delusion disorder |
| **Flies** in | **Folie** à deux |
| **Pairs make me** | **Paraphrenia** |
| **Paranoid** | **Paranoia** |

For some special **paranoid** conditions there is:

### Hypochondriac Fergi Declares Othello is Crap

| | |
|---|---|
| **Hypochondria** | Monosymptomatic **hypochondria**cal psychosis (MHP) |
| **Fergi** | **Fregoli** syndrome |
| **Declares** | **De Cler**ambault syndrome |
| **Othello** | **Othello** |
| **Crap** | **Capgras** |

**SWOT BOX**

In **monosymptomatic hypochondriacal psychosis** the patient is convinced there is a physical cause of complaint and 'gathers evidence' for it. **De Clerambault** syndrome is also known as *erotomania* and is the belief of one person that another person (usually unattainable) loves them intensely. People affected by **Fregoli syndrome** believe many different people are actually the same person who changes appearance or is in disguise. The **Othello delusion** is one in which there is a belief that one's partner is unfaithful. In **Capgras syndrome**, there is a belief that a familiar person has been replaced by an exact double or an imposter.

# Depression

Seven things to look out for in depression:

## 7 As of depression

**A**nhedonia
**A**ppetite loss
**A**nergia
**A**M waking
**A**menorrhoea
**A**sexual (decreased **libido**)
**A**ffective disorder

There are eight things in this scheme of DESPAIRS:[1]

## DESPAIRS

| | |
|---|---|
| **D** | **Depressed mood or disinterest** |
| **E** | **Energy loss, TATT (tired all the time)** |
| **S** | **Sleep disturbed** |
| **P** | **Pessimism, hopelessness, worthlessness** |
| **A** | **Appetite and weight change** |
| **I** | **Impaired concentration** |
| **R** | **Retardation or agitation** |
| **S** | **Suicidal ideas or recurrent thoughts** |

1 From Kendrick T. (2003) *The New Generalist* **1**(2).

> 🎓 **SWOT BOX**
>
> The syndrome of depression comprises the first symptom + at least four others + significant functional impairment for > 2 weeks (preferably several weeks).

# Mental state exam

### Mad Is Pat?

| | |
|---|---|
| **M** | **Mood** |
| **A** | **Appearance** |
| **D** | **Diet (appetite)/Depression** |
| **I** | **Insight** |
| **S** | **Speech** |
| **P** | **Perceptual (sensory)** |
| **A** | **Appearance/Anxiety** |
| **T** | **Thoughts** |
| **?** | **Memory** (concentration) |

## *Alternative*

'**Pam's BMI**' stands for: Thoughts, Orientation, Perceptual, Appearance, Mood, Speech, Behaviour, Memory, Insight.

# Schizophrenia

**Classification** of is as follows:

### Cats Simply Hate Parrots

| | |
|---|---|
| **Cats** | **Catatonic** |
| **Simply** | **Simple** |
| **Hate** | **Hebephrenic** |
| **Parrots** | **Paranoid** |

The **acute features** are:

## SHADI

S           **Stress/Stimulation (precipitated by)**
H          **Hallucinations**
A          **Affect is incongruent**
D         **Deletions of thought**
I           **Interference with thinking**

The **chronic features** include age, disorientation, lack of volition, loosening of associations (formal thought disorder), apathy, poverty of (poor) speech and thought, blunting of affect, deteriorating social conduct (e.g. swearing in public or at staff), social withdrawal and underactivity (slowness). They are all covered in the rude poem!

 **NAUGHTY BIT**

To a dizzy young violinist called Shadi
'Stop losing your socks, you're all apathy!'
Poor Shadi was blunt
Doctor you are a ****!
Thus withdrawing, we slowed down entirely.

The key to this verse is:

| | |
|---|---|
| **Dizzy** | **Disorientated** |
| **Young** | **Age** |
| **Violinist** | **Voli**tion |
| **Losing** your socks | **Loosening** of associations |
| **Apathy** | **Apathy** |
| **Poor** | **Poverty** of speech and thought |
| **Blunt** | **Blunt**ing of affect |
| **Withdrawing** | **Withdrawal** |
| **Slowed** | **Slow**ness and underactivity |

# Chapter Twelve

# RADIOLOGY

## Chest X-ray

The mediastinal contours seen on chest X-ray (from top to bottom) are shown below.

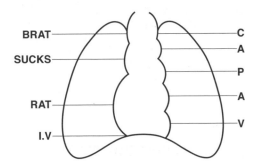

For the right, use:

### Brat Sucks Rats I.V.

| | |
|---|---|
| **Brat** | **Brachiocephalic vein** |
| **Sucks** | **SVC (superior vena cava)** |
| **RAT**s | **Right ATrium** |
| I.V. | **IVC (inferior vena cava)** |

And for the left:

**LAP–AV**

| | |
|---|---|
| **L** | **Left subclavian** |
| **A** | **Aorta** |
| **P** | **Pulmonary artery** |
| **A** | **Atrium** |
| **V** | **Ventricle** |

# Emphysema

The hyperinflated chest X-ray gives the mediastinum the typical 'strung chicken' appearance. It is:

### The Strung Up Chicken of Emphysema

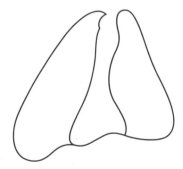

# Congestive cardiac failure

With congestive heart failure the chest X-ray has a bat's-wing appearance, and this is known as:

### The Bat Signal

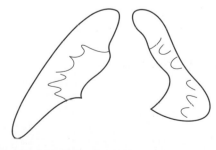

# Crohn's disease

You need to know the following characteristics features of Crohn's on **X-ray**. This one was contributed anonymously.

| | |
|---|---|
| C | **Cobblestone appearance of mucosa** |
| R | **Rose-thorn ulcers** |
| O | **Obstruction of bowel** |
| H | **Hyperplasia of mesenteric lymph nodes** |
| N | **Narrowing of lumen** |
| S | **Skip lesions (Sarcoid foci/Steatorrhoea)** |

# Vertebral fractures

When looking for spinal fractures check for the elephant's skull – you can easily imagine two eyes and a nose. If you cannot clearly see two eyes and a nose on a particular vertebra then it is likely to be fractured.

### The Elephant's Skull

**Can't see two eyes and a nose? Consider fracture**

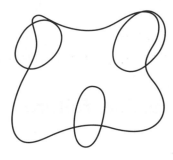

# SECTION III

## STUDY TIPS AND MEMORY BITS

# Chapter Thirteen

# MAKING YOUR OWN MNEMONICS

The Big Secret of mnemonics is to make it fun – using both hemispheres of the brain plus an element of fun engages your mind. While you are working on your mnemonic you are likely to be focused on the subject, regardless of how well the actual mnemonic works.

Rule one is to keep your mnemonics short and sweet (e.g. 'Mighty Ape' for the MT–AP sequence of heart sounds is quick and easy and obvious). Too many long anagram-type mnemonics are limited because they presuppose that you will know what the first letter stands for! So, rather than having mnemonics consisting of just several initial letters, aim for a multilevel approach. For instance, look at the *first two, or even three letters*, and try to phrase a word or sentence that is relevant to the subject matter – 'Those Giant Gonads Prolong the Action' tells you at least the first two or three letters of the names of the anterior pituitary hormones, and the phrase is also in context with the topic, as well as being humorous.

*Patterns* are very important too. Consider 'Hammer Toe Is Proximal To Mallet Toe'– well, this is true, and they are also in alphabetical order. Similarly, ' Two Lungs and One Heart' uses a pattern in the structure to relate to the location of beta-2 receptors on the lungs (2 lungs) and of beta-1 receptors on the heart (1 heart).

So if something isn't sticking in your head, check for any patterns or letters or sounds that help you remember it. Consider Weber's test and Rinne's test: Weber's test involves touching the tuning fork in the midline, and of course the first letter (W) of the word Weber has a midline – unlike the 'R' in Rinne's test. That's an easy way to distinguish them, and you'll never confuse the two again.

Rude mnemonics can be very funny – but use them sparingly or you may forget who is doing what to whom and with what!

Listen out for any sounds that may give clues, as in the verse used to learn features of chronic schizophrenia in the psychiatry chapter. Look for visual clues, too, such as the fact that the lower case letter 'b' looks like an upside down digit 'q' – hence, haemophilia B is due to lack of factor q.

It is always a good idea to write your mnemonics down in your own notebook (or in the spaces available in this book), together with your own explanatory notes if you want, so that you can scan them rapidly the night before an exam.

Even if your mnemonic is not helpful to other people, it will have been useful to you – the act of generating a mnemonic means you are concentrating on the subject at hand.

And remember – *mnemonics* do help, but *fun* helps even more. Enjoy!

In the next chapter we introduce the 'memory training' concepts of link and association.

# Chapter Fourteen

# LEARNING WITH THE LINK

*In the first place, association*
Harry Lorayne and Jerry Lucas *(The Memory Book)*

Association is the process that links the new fact or word you want to learn with some information that you already know – numbers, the alphabet, members of your family, your bedroom, etc.

We know that the nature of brain pathways are such that any word or thought can link you to a myriad of other words (see your neurology textbooks). In fact, your brain works in a non-linear fashion, like a mind-map.

Take for instance the word 'chocolate' – many mental associations can come to mind immediately if you channel your thoughts in this direction. Almost instantaneously you will generate hundreds of thoughts, ideas, words, connotations, mental images, memories and so on. And you do it all while being totally relaxed and laid back about the whole experience!

So if your brain already works this way, naturally, why not make use of it to deliberately associate new facts to things you already know?

You can repeat a fact to yourself until your brain gets the message and creates a link in a random way (like, how long will that take!). Or you can make it easier.

There is nothing new about association – the technique was used by the ancient Greeks to memorize key words in their long orations. They would take a mental tour around their homes, having already associated key concepts to objects they already knew. After all, you remember where your bed is and what your bathroom looks like. The phrase 'In the first place' is said to come from this practise. This is the 'loci' memory system (spatial mnemonics) and it is still used by speech-makers and memory experts (and for example, is great for learning the Krebs cycle – see below).

Making associations deliberately is achieved using mental pictures. You need to exercise your imagination by producing vivid and exaggerated pictures in your mind, evoking strong imaginary emotions and which are as ridiculous and out of place as possible. If you have made it this far you already have the skills to learn a few 'advanced' memory tricks!

For instance, if a pigeon flew over your head yesterday at lunchtime, chances are you won't even remember it. But if an elephant with a striped hockey stick and yellow polka-dot boxer shorts flew over your head you would most likely remember the image for the rest of your life! You may also remember what day it was and what you were doing at the time.

So, to learn a short list, you can mentally 'link' one item to the next. Make your imaginary pictures extreme, exaggerated, ridiculous, bold, funny and outrageous. (It's okay – it's all in your head!)

*The golden rule* is to ask yourself 'If it happened in real life is it something I would always remember?'. For example, if Martians landed in your back yard. You see, you can make it up and it will be just as memorable.

# Chapter Fifteen

# THE POWER OF THE PEG

## ...and conquering those cranial nerves

Having delved into the world of making associations with extreme pictures, we can try simple 'peg', which enables you to learn lists easily and reliably in and out of sequence. To do this you have to know how to count up to, say, 12. (Peg systems do exist that go up into the thousands!)

First, spend the next 60 seconds memorizing the following numbered list:

1. run
2. shoe
3. tree
4. door
5. hive
6. sticks
7. heaven
8. gate
9. dine (or 'line')
10. hen
11. level crossing (or 'leaven')
12. elves (or 'Twelfth Night')

Done it? Here we have learnt a system for using *images* to code for *numbers*, in order to make visualization easy. We begin associating our list to the twelve pairs of cranial nerves. You don't have to use my suggestions – your own will work much better.

- Cranial nerve I is the **olfactory**. Imagine say, an *oil factory* (or *oil refinery* or perhaps an *oil drilling platform*). These are 'substitute' words to help you remember the word 'olfactory'. Using substitutes facilitates visualization of vague terms. So the *oil factory* will be your analogy for the first nerve. Meanwhile you know that a substitute word for 1 is RUN. Now add movement – see, for instance, this *oil factory* growing enormous legs, like an ostrich or a dinosaur, and *running* down your street, as fast as it's huge gangling, creaking bulk will allow. Close your eyes for a moment to let that picture crystallize clearly in your mind. Involve all of your senses; *smell* that crude oil (it is the first nerve after all!). *See* splodges of oil being shaken off and landing all over the place. *Feel* the ground shudder with each step. We have now associated 1 with *olfactory*. Easy enough?

- So let us travel to 2 which, in our system, transposes to SHOE. Cranial nerve II or 2 is the **optic** and 2 codes for 'shoe'. Visualize wearing *shoes* instead of *glasses* (optics), or maybe smashing a pair of *optics* by stamping on them with your favourite, newest, most expensive shoes. See the vivid image, and now exaggerate it beyond belief – make those optics shatter into millions of pieces which fly up and gather into a whirlpool of whizzing optics while your shoe continues on relentlessly…

- The IIIrd nerve is the **oculomotor**. Imagine your TREE with motorized branches, and at the end of each branch is an *eye* (*oculus*). The eyes are clicking and whirring on those motorized branches, all focusing and staring at you – hundreds of motorized eyes looking straight into yours…and yet you have an unusual feeling of well being as you realize these are your creation, entirely safe within your mind's *oculus*, with you in total control. Make the motorized branches dance and whirl as they click and spin. Got the picture? If not, make up another one!

- Nerve IV is the **trochlear**. We use DOOR to represent the number 4. Not just *any* door, but one that is meaningful to you – e.g. your own front door or that of somebody close to you. A substitute word for trochlear may be *truck* or *trog* (or even a pulley if you know that *trochilia* is Greek for a pulley). The possibilities are now limitless! Whatever you decide, make the image bright, bold, and noisy and exaggerated in every sense.

- The substitute word for 5 is HIVE. Nerve V is the **trigeminal**. You may for instance visualize an enormous hive, but instead of bees or wasps imagine of lots of precious *gems* buzzing around the hive; see them whizzing in and out and flying about your ears as they sparkle and shine. Make it so ridiculous and surreal that *if you saw it in real life you would remember it forever*. Alternatively you can use the word *gem*ini for trigeminal, as well as, say, triplets (instead of twins) and then link those *tri*plets to the bee hive. Use whatever forms your association in the easiest most memorable way.

- Number 6 transposes to STICKS. The VIth cranial nerve is the **abducens**. You can use a simple picture such as *abducting* your arms with a big *stick*, although in this case make the picture really vivid.

- The number 7 is HEAVEN and the VIIth cranial nerve is the **facial** nerve. You can graphically visualise many faces, including your own, falling down from the sky (heaven). See in detail the expressions on these millions of faces as they keep falling down relentlessly – large faces, small faces… Also try imagining cloud-shaped faces floating in the sky, perhaps some are laughing, some are frowning, and some are smiling, etc.

- We now need to link the number 8 (GATF) to the **vestibulocochlear** nerve (VIII) to a possible mnemonic lists, such as movies you know well…or watch as many movies as you can that you love, or videos of sporting events and finals. So see a gate in your mind, *not* just *any* gate, but a gate of importance to you, such as your own front gate, or perhaps one on a building you admire. Alternatively you may see a *giant ear* in place of the *gate* which you have to push aside in order to get through the gate.

- Let's link 9 (DINE) to the **glossopharyngeal** nerve. Although you should have the hang of it by now, one suggestion is of a giant *pharynx* being dined upon – at a very *glossy* dinner party. Give the giant pharynx a good dose of pharyngitis. *Hear* it sound hoarse and make it *look* very sore and phlegmy.

- Number 10 is 'hen'. See an enormous hen perhaps laying an egg – make the hen look suitably *vague* for the **vagus** (or dress it up like a *magus*). Maybe a hen on the cover of *Vogue* magazine would work for you. Or whatever…

- For number 11 you could instead visualize a 'level crossing' for this number. Cranial nerve **XI** is the **accessory** nerve. You decide which type of *accessories* to use here.

- Number 12 rhymes with 'elve'. Imagine a dozen elves with giant *tongues* hanging out. Perhaps they are all experiencing *hypos* because they are unable to eat because of the size of their giant tongues. This should be sufficient to remind you of the **hypoglossal** nerve.

IMPORTANT: Now run through those silly images two or three more times during the next couple of minutes. So now we have:

- run – olfactory (*see* the mental picture you made)
- shoe – optic
- tree – oculomotor

- door – trochlear
- hive – trigeminal
- sticks – abducens
- heaven – facial
- gate – vestibulocochlear
- dine (or line) – glossopharyngeal
- lien – vagus
- level crossing (or leaven) – accessory
- elves – hypoglossal.

Run through this list, from the top to the bottom, in your head a couple more times, then do it backwards.

We are ready for a test!

Which is the seventh nerve? (Think of number seven; see the picture that you imagined, e.g. faces in the sky. Note how you link this picture to what represents a…facial nerve. And you know it is the seventh nerve. *How cool is that?*)

Okay, now try these:

- Which is the eleventh nerve?
- Which cranial nerve is the oculomotor?
- Which cranial nerve is in the abducens?
- Which is the first cranial nerve?

Looks like you've got the hang of it! Incidentally, even if you didn't stop and review things along the way *as instructed* (and I'm pretty sure you didn't) you would still have got most of these correct!

Congratulations you now know the cranial nerves *in* and out of order, and you know the number assigned to them also, in and out of order too! You did this with ease and loads of fun. Review them a few more times now in order to cement them into your long-term memory.

*Note:* After using this several times you will no longer require the actual mnemonics.

*Imagination is more important than knowledge*
Albert Einstein

# Chapter Sixteen

# SPATIAL MNEMONICS

*Krebs' cycle in your kitchen*

Sometimes described as the 'loci' (Greek *locus* meaning place) system of memory, this was used for thousands of years as a memory aid. It fell out of favour with the arrival of the printing press. The first documented source is from Cicero who described how in 516 BC the poet Simonides escaped a disaster that destroyed the building he was dining in along with many other public figures. By recalling where they had been seated, he named all of the deceased.

This powerful methods uses the locations of fixed reference objects to learn information by associating and *linking* what you already know (e.g. what your bedroom looks like) to what you wish to learn (e.g. the biochemical cycles).

Not too dissimilar are the oral memory traditions of many cultures whereby major events from a particular year (e.g. a flood or a storm) are linked to other happenings. Frances Yates gives a very detailed account in *The Art of Memory* (Chicago: University of Chicago Press Chicago, 1966).

Once you learn how with the example given below you can apply these techniques to anything you wish.

## Spatial mnemonics in seven minutes

Link the new fact or word you *need* to learn (e.g. the Krebs cycle) with information that you *already remember* (e.g. your kitchen, your journey to college, members of your family, your bedroom, etc.). This process of *linking* helps us associate one bit of info to another. On p. 56 you learned the actions of beta-blockers using parts of your own body to link the facts to. We earlier discussed making those extreme, exaggerated mental links and associations.

*Ask yourself: If it happened in real life, is it something I would always remember?*

For instance, you might conjure up a huge, smelly, red rhinoceros kissing your nose. Whatever you make it up should be just as memorable.

# KK's six steps to spatial mnemonics

1. **Start at a fixed point** – e.g. the DOOR or entrance.
2. **Go clockwise** around the room (or from beginning to end if it is a journey or route that you are using).
3. **Link the chunk of information wish to learn** to the object you will always remember (whether it is your bedroom door or kitchen fridge). If you can remember where these fixed reference points are, then you can succeed at spatial mnemonics. Make your mental associations extreme, exaggerated, silly, ridiculous, dramatic and *always* over-the-top. You may also add some movement or action (remember the rhinoceros?) to the scene.
4. **Finish back at the door** – our starting point – so you know that we have completed the topic.
5. **Review** by walking around the room (this can be done *virtually*, as in the example below, but it's probably better if you can actually be in the same place). Imagine your mnemonic unfolding in front of you. Review a few times in other locations, like the bus stop and hairdressers. Make day-dreaming productive!
6. **Revise** by making notes (e.g. write it down, tabulate, mind-map it, use rough sketches or diagrams). Closer to exam time, revise from these notes you made on the mnemonic! Teaching your friends the day before helps you to revise (you don't have to mention you are using spatial mnemonics if you want to show off – Beware though! Your superb recall may make you less popular!).

*Your imagination…is worth more than you imagine*
After French writer Louis Aragon

*Imagination is more important than knowledge*
Albert Einstein

# Spatial mnemonic for the Krebs cycle

Here is the tricarboxylic acid (TCA) or Krebs cycle – try it out in your kitchen!

| | |
|---|---|
| Oxaloacetate | (4 carbon) |
| Citrate | (6 carbon) |
| Isocitrate | (6 carbon) |
| Ketoglutarate | (5 carbon) |
| Succinyl co-A | (4 carbon) |
| Succinate | (4 carbon) |
| Fumarate | (4 carbon) |
| Malate | (4 carbon) |

- **Start at a fixed point.** We will start at the kitchen door. Think of your chosen kitchen door. What colour and texture is it? What is it made of? Wood or glass? It may be just a doorway.
- Now link door to the title i.e. Krebs cycle. We can use a *substitute* word like 'crabs'. So imagine a huge mighty crab guarding the kitchen entrance, snapping away at you with its mighty pincers. Notice the bright colours and contours of its shell…
- Did of you notice I emphasized a mighty crab? This is because Krebs occurs in the *mito*chondrion. Just threw in an extra mnemonic for the same price. Get the picture? Good. Now make it more vivid and *turn up the volume!*
- Working our way clockwise on our mental tour around the room, the next object is the cooker. For this demonstration, we need to link **oxaloacetate** (four-carbon compound) to the cooker – how about an *ox* on the cooker? Imagine an ox is sitting on it…oxaloacetate…Wrap it in two layers of *acetate* so the two carbons – acetate – are then added. And a cooker has four hobs so emphasize that.
- Now link one of the cupboards…to **citrate**. We continue the story by opening the cupboard, from which *citrus* juice floods out, making our eye sore – **isocitrate**? So far so good – stay with me. We *blow* the juice off our sore eyes, hence blowing off our $CO_2$, which *loses us a carbon*, the next item – the *cat* eating *glue* in the microwave – *alpha-***ketoglutarate**. You *dive* (= five) to save the cat and blow it out and *lose another carbon* as $CO_2$ – taking you to the sink.
- *Sucking coal* in the *sink*? Yep, it's **succinyl co-A**, for sure.
- And next to that is the dishwasher – where you are sucking an *8*-ball. To make it **succinate**.
- Then there is **fumarate** – the *fuming* kettle.

- Then **malate** – *mole ate* the bin.
- And after that, we are back at the beginning, in the doorway, with the *mighty crab*.

Congratulations! You have just completed your first spatial mnemonic, memorizing the Krebs cycle (*including* the numbers of carbon atoms) and you did it in somebody else's virtual kitchen! If any steps are unclear, go back and reinforce them. The technique generally works better with your own mnemonics in your own environment, where your own belongings are more familiar – think just how much more powerful this would be in a kitchen you are familiar with.

| What we need to learn | Fixed reference points (examples as given above) | Your kitchen's fixed reference points (fill in as you sit in the nearest kitchen) | Your spatial mnemonic (e.g. a mighty crab guarding the door) | Examples as given above |
|---|---|---|---|---|
| Krebs cycle steps | Door/entrance | Door/entrance (start here and work clockwise) | | Mighty crab guarding door |
| Oxaloacetate | Cooker | | | Ox on cooker with four hobs, wrapped acetate × 2 |
| Citrate | Cupboards | | | Citrus fruits |
| Isocitrate | Opened the cupboards | | | Made your eye sore |
| Alpha-ketoglutarate | Microwave | | | Cat eating glue in microwave |
| Succinyl Co-A | Sink | | | Sucking coal in sink |
| Succinate | Dishwasher | | | Sucking an 8-ball |
| Fumarate | Kettle | | | Fuming kettle |
| Malate | Bin | | | Mole ate the bin |
| Back to beginning | Doorway | | | |

# Chapter Seventeen

# REVISE AT THE MOVIES!

## More links and loci

In the last section you learned memory consists of linking what we *want* to know with what we *already* know – and as you can associate anything to anything else, it is possible to use your favourite movies, soap or sporting event to revise. People often remember their favourite movie or sporting event in remarkable detail. Why not put that to good use? Make use of movies, events and football teams that you already know by heart. The more detail you know, the more facts you can associate into your key scenes, characters, players, sportsmen, and so on.

We will explore how to make use of a memory we already have to learn something we need for our exams!

I use as our example *The Wizard of Oz* (by L. Frank Baum) on the assumption that it is likely to be familiar to all or most of our readers. (Hey stop complaining – or I'll make you use *The Sound of Music*!) If you somehow have managed *not* to see this film then go and watch it now – it is essential for your revision!

Okay, you already know how to link memories consciously – by associating them to something you already know, by exaggerated use of your imagination. (If you don't already know how, then go and read the last chapter, you skiver! Honestly!)

So what to learn? As an example, just for the heck of it, why not learn the peripheral somatosensory system pain and temperature pathway? As these pathways are quite awkward to learn you may as well get it out of the way now.

Of course, you can use *any other* list or topic you wish; this book is your willing slave, after all – not the other way round! Here goes...

# The peripheral somatosensory system pain and temperature pathway

- **Receptors** are in the dermis/epidermis of skin (arranged in overlapping **dermatomes**).
- Sensory neurons travel to the **dorsal root ganglion** (a few branches will travel up or down a segment and enter the dorsal horn at a different level – this allows **overlap**).
- The nerve synapses in the **dorsal horn** of the spinal cord.
- The second (postganglionic) neuron now **crosses over** to the contralateral side in the **ventral white matter**.
- Then it ascends in the lateral white matter.
- Some short **secondary internuncial neurons** – they connect with motor neurons to form the **reflex arc.** By the way 'internuncial' refers to 'linking' neurons – which is exactly what you are doing now.
- Back to the collection of crossed fibres – the **lateral spinothalamic tract.**
- They travel to the **thalamus** where they synapse in the **ventral posterolateral nucleus** (VPL).
- Tertiary neurons now go to the **postcentral gyrus** (area 3, 1, 2) of the cortex – the main somatic sensory area of the brain.

I have selected a few key words here – once we have a group of key words we can begin constructing a mnemonic-based memory aid.

Back to *The Wizard of Oz*! We need the key events from the story. Briefly:

- Dorothy lives on farm in Kansas with dog, Toto
- House is blown away up into a tornado
- House crash-lands in Oz
- Munchkins
- Glinda the good witch enters
- Glinda gives Dorothy pair of ruby slippers
- Dorothy follows the yellow brick road
- Meets the scarecrow who wants a brain
- Meets the tin woodman who needs oiling and a heart

- Meets the cowardly lion
- Have nice snoozy time in field of scarlet poppies (quite advanced, I thought, for a kiddie's movie, but then maybe I am showing my age!)
- Emerald city – wear emerald glasses
- Meet the wizard...
- ...who sends them off to defeat wicked witch of the West
- Travel through dark enchanted forest
- Carried to the horrible witch by winged monkeys
- Dorothy melts witch with bucket of water
- Oz turns out to be fake wizard with big balloon
- Dorothy clicks heels together to get home

So now all you need to do is link *what* you need to know with what you *already* know about the *Wizard of Oz*. I have put in one or two suggestions, but now *you* have to do some of the dream work – it's much more fun than normal work. Once you have learned the principle, you can use it with other movies or soap operas, the FA Cup final or World Cup 1966, or whatever.

| What you know already | Facts you need to learn | Dream work (my suggestions – but make your own notes) |
| --- | --- | --- |
| KANSAS, FARM | Pain and temperatures | Very hot on farm. Exaggerate the image beyond belief! |
| TORNADO | Start with PAIN and temperature in the dermis | Tornado blows off all of Toto's and Dorothy's dermis and epidermis |
| CRASH LAND | Dorsal root ganglion | Crash on back of (dorsum) of a gang of Munchkins? Make the pictures vivid, put in sound and colour and sensations |
| MUNCHKINS | | |
| GLINDA/RUBY SLIPPERS | Branches overlapping up/down a level | So many slippers that slippers are overlapping with her shoes |
| YELLOW BRICK ROAD | Synapse, dorsal horn | If you haven't read the previous chapter by this stage you may be a little lost – go back now! |
| SCARECROW | Crossing over | Make your own images, outrageous and whacky ones |
| TINMAN | | |
| LION | | The rule is one mnemonic per movie! |

| SCARLET POPPY FIELD | Ascending in the lateral white matter | Etc. ... | |
|---|---|---|---|
| EMERALD CITY | Short neurons form the reflex arc | | |
| WIZARD OF OZ | Lateral spinothalamic tract | | |
| DARK FOREST | Thalamus | | |
| WINGED MONKEYS | Synapse in VPL | | |
| WITCH MELTING | Postcentral gyrus | | |
| BOGUS WIZARD FLIES OFF IN BALLOON | Near the central fissure | | |
| CLICK HEELS THREE TIMES | Area 3, 1, 2 | | Dorothy counts 3-1-2 as she clicks her heels, but she's a bit dizzy and gets the numbers out of order |

# Homework (dreamwork)!

Now that you are getting the hang of it:

• Go watch a movie…one that you know and love really well. One in which you always remember the main scenes or characters. Being able to pause the scenes makes it even easier.
• Make a list of other memorable events you know really well like weddings, football matches, hockey finals, etc.
• Try using routes too, maybe your route to college – you may have done it hundreds of times and know it backwards (this is the loci system again).
• Try making lists of other things you know, perhaps of your flatmates, characters in your bridge club, or whatever.
• Pick a few topics in which sequences are important and dig out the *key words* – this is one of the most important stages because it makes you *summarize* and *review* as you do so. And you'll remember that summarizing and reviewing are the two most important revision skills, regardless of *how* you do them.
• Make a table like that above, and jot down in rough pencil your mental imagery. Or you can use a mind-map.
• When revision time comes you will only need to revise your jotted down notes on your mnemonic and not pile through pages of text – a serious time-saver for 'night-before' revision!

Enjoy!

# Chapter Eighteen

# MOTIVATIONAL BITS, QUIPS AND STUDY TIPS

A potpourri of thoughts, ideas, musings and wisdom, ancient and modern, together with a soupçon of solidly useful study tips to see you on your way…

Suddenly the euphoria of being at university is gone; there is an eerie silence in the air; where once there was laughter and milling throngs all around is despair. And worst of all is the weird sensation that even though you are surrounded by hundreds of other people, you are almost alone…Yep, it's exam season again!

Well, like I said, *almost* alone – now is the time you find out who your friends really are – and you will have discovered that this little book is up there with the best of them!

So strap yourself into that chair/couch/bed, put the kettle on and prepare to share the wisdom of some of the world's finest thinkers – and as you meld in this way remember that you too are amongst them!

*The surest way to be late is have plenty of time*
Leo Kennedy

# How common *is* common?

Remember this if you're ever stuck for figures:

| | |
|---|---|
| **1 : 30** | **Common** |
| **1 : 300** | **Uncommon** |
| **1 : 300** | **Rare** |

# Regular breaks and time outs

Have regular breaks! This is evidence-based folks – you retain more and work more productively if you have sensible rest or gaps during your challenging schedule.

Say for a full day of study:

- Start off with breaks of 10–20 minutes each hour when you are fresh.
- Be flexible with your breaks – with experience your own body will tell you what feels right.
- Then as the hours pass by and your interest starts flagging, in order to keep you studying efficiently, you may need to increase the break times.
- So by the evening you may have half an hour of swotting followed by a half-hour break.
- Before you start your break, run through what you have just done, in your mind, for a few seconds only – so you rapidly skim through main headings and points at high speed.
- When you come back from your break, rapidly skim through the stuff you did previously, in your mind's eye, again for a few seconds – this sets you up quickly to get back into 'mode'.

This way in any 12-hour period you will get several hours' productive revision done. Working flat out without a break only gives you useful revision for the first few hours; after that you become tired, possibly lose interest, and your learning starts flagging. Twelve hours straight without a break is very inefficient compared with the same period with realistic, generous and regular breaks.

   Remember to eat too.

# Buddies

Hopefully you can surround yourself with a good group of revision buddies. It helps to teach each other different parts of the syllabus (hugely time saving). You will have your own individual strategy of course.

# Caffeine

Certainly extremely useful as a mild stimulant – but beware of overdoing it as it can only give you so much of a lift before the shakes start, and diuresis (not helpful to you during exams) and, even worse, diarrhoea and wind (not helpful to the person in the chair behind you).

Sleep deprivation is also unhelpful. And remember that caffeine may stay in your system for hours, so even when you do sleep it will reduce the overall quality of that sleep and may result in that 'why am I tired all the time if I am having loads of caffeine?' syndrome. Be good to yourself. And set realistic goals.

# Patterns

Students have used patterned representations for years to learn particular syndromes, for example for hypothyroidism, acromegaly, respiratory failure (pink puffers and blue bloaters) and so on. This includes photographs of rare patients with 'classical' signs, caricatures, drawings and – best of all – your personal memories of particular case studies. Medicine is after all much to do with 'pattern matching' and it will help during revision and self-testing also (although remember these are at best generalizations and their main purpose is to get you through tomorrow's exam).

# Goal-setting

- Define your study goals/amounts/times before you start.
- Give yourself *realistic* targets – learn *smarter*. Time is limited (both for you and your swotty neighbour). If it won't help you pass, then ignore! As Emerson said 'Life is too short…!'.
- Define your *break times*. A count-down timer is useful and can be found on most digital watches, microwaves and kitchen appliances.
- *Allow for 2 minutes' overview at the beginning of each session and 5 minutes' review at the end.*
- Decide what you will learn *now* and what you will cover *later* – when and if you have the time. This is called *prioritizing* your resources and it is a skill that is especially important to doctors.
- Define goals for the session, the day, the term, the year – or even set lifelong targets. The use of goals and targets has permeated all walks of life, from fiscal to political, motivational and self-development for the simple reason that goal-setting *works*! Write down your goals, aims and objectives.
- However, if your dominant thoughts are about a football match, a movie, or going out – good news! *It is still possible to 'mnemonic' these events by associating them with the facts you wish to learn.*

- Fill your thoughts with images and visions of yourself making the *exam* suffer for using up so much of your time…. Aim for an elegantly detached matter-of-fact state whereby there is just enough adrenaline and sympathetic activity to keep you alert and interested.

 **The SMART goals are**

S   pecific and simple
M   easurable and meaningful
A   ll relevant areas
R   ealistic and Responsible
T   imed toward what you want

- According to Edison, genius is 1% inspiration and 99% perspiration. Many of your colleagues are saying that they have not done any work. What they really mean is that they have not done as much as they would like – and have actually done more than they realize, or are prepared to admit!
- This is a common phenomenon in the medical schools' game because the selection process seems to pick out many pathological perfectionists…they could *never* have done enough work and rely on denial as a bizarre motivational strategy.
- This is fine because different people work in different ways. Your task is to recognize this and accept it. Nobody knows as much as you think they do – and you know more than you realize!
- Remember – nobody knows everything. Walter Mondale said 'If you think you understand everything that is going on, you are hopelessly confused'. Make your learning efficient and ecological, and pay particular attention to your learning environment.

# Environment

Learning is a process by which your brain makes certain neurological connections. Learning is a process by which your brain makes certain neurological connections. Everything happening to you at the time you learn adds a few sub-branches to that particular connection in your neural network (see your neurology texts).

So if you are doped up on caffeine while revising, your brain remembers that too. When you need to reproduce the information in your exam with no caffeine in your bloodstream, your brain will find it that much harder to access the facts you need. This is why psychologists describe learning as being 'state-specific'.

In other words, aim to match every aspect of your environment – including biochemical factors – to simulate as near as possible the exam conditions. If possible, you can even revise the subject in the room you will be taking the exam in. If this is not possible, then you can use different rooms for different subjects (so that thinking of a specific room, what it looks and feels like, will act as a memory jogger). This also helps reduce confusion between different subjects.

(You may have heard about students who could only pass exams while having a raised blood ethanol level, who are useless while sober! Now you know why.)

Try to make sure your blood levels of caffeine and glucose are the same as what they will be during the exam. If certain music helps you to remember but you are then not allowed to wear personal stereos during the exam, beware! (If there is no other option, listen to your music on the morning of the exam). Take whatever sensible and logical steps you can – then go for it!

# Go for it

*What you can do, or dream you can...begin it*
*Boldness has genius, power and magic in it*

Goethe

*Make it so!*
Captain Jean-Luc Picard (in *Star Trek: The Next Generation*)

*People wish to learn to swim*
*and at the same time to keep one foot on the ground*

Marcel Proust

# Goodness

*To the good, be good*
*To the bad be good too*
*In order to make them good as well*

The He Zhizhang, Tang Dynasty

*The good is the beautiful*

Lysis (Plato)

*If you cannot speak good of someone, be silent*

Reported by Bukhari

# Internet

The Internet is a huge resource of study tips, notes, mnemonics and other people's PowerPoint™ presentations (ppt's). Just beware of the validity of this information and also the fact that it may be out of date, or just plain wrong. Double-check and cross-reference the material unless you are very sure.

# Key facts

You are aware of the concept of key words and key facts or phrases – to put it simply, those facts that will give you *marks* in the exam. Once you have gained an understanding of a topic, don't spend time learning anything unless it can be classed as directly relevant to obtaining exam marks. Once exams and assessments are no longer an issue you can, of course, learn as many irrelevant facts as you wish! And have a good laugh about it. Even better, laugh all the way through your revision too.

# Laughter

> When the first baby laughed for the first time, the laugh broke into a thousand pieces and they all went skipping about, and that was the beginning of fairies
>
> *Peter Pan*

# Maps and territories

> The map is not the territory
>
> Alfred Korzybski

# Mind-maps

*Use mind-maps.* Invented by Tony Buzan decades ago, these are surprisingly underused. Many of you will have come across them at school. Mind-maps are especially useful for previewing a topic at the start of a study session, reviewing it at the end, and for making essay and project plans.

They are very useful if you are doing an exam with lots of sections or written parts. You start off several mind-maps, one for each section. Then you start writing your answers. As you write, the earlier questions serve as memory joggers and ideas will come for the later parts. You can immediately jot these down onto your other mind-maps.

If you attempt to answer a question you know nothing about, doodling with a mind-map can extract some answers from the inner recesses of your unconscious mind! Here's how to do one:

- Start in the centre, using plenty of colours and icons, images and doodles all the way through your mind-map.
- Collect your key words and add them to the map.
- Connect each key word with a line to the central idea and also to other related areas of the map.
- Use thinner lines as you get further away from the centre.
- Use your own style.
- Remember, other people's mind-maps tend to be less useful than the ones you created yourself.

# Morning before

Okay, so you're up, ideally having had a few hours of sleep to let yesterday's revision sink into your longish-term memory. Now have breakfast! (Unless, of course, you have done all of your learning on an empty stomach – see 'Environment' above).

If you used caffeine during your revision then have one cup of whatever you used, now. Skim through your cards, summarized notes, mind-maps and *mnemonics*. Reinforce the material you have previously covered.

It makes sense to have at least an hour of mental relaxation just before the exam to let everything sink in and assimilate, allowing your neurotransmitter levels to recharge. You will need them at their peak to blitz these exams.

# Night before

It is usually better to get a few hours of quality sleep the night before – the rare exception is when you only have a single exam to do and really have done no preparation whatsoever. Having worked efficiently with plenty of breaks (see 'Breaks' and 'Environment') you should be tired enough to get to sleep. The day/night before is usually when your mnemonics are most helpful (that is why we have made this book a portable size).

However, if you **have** a string of exams to sit over a period of several days simply staying up all night will turn you into a zomboid amnesiac, staring blankly at your exam paper.

While you sleep your mind keeps working, sorting and assimilating what you have learned. If you stay awake all night, learning lots of last-minute minutiae, you will certainly remember what you have just read in the last two hours or so (short-term memory) but are likely to have forgotten much of the earlier stuff. You decide if the trade-off is worth it (very occasionally it is).

# Patients and preparation

*The best preparation for tomorrow is to do today's work superbly well*

*To study medicine without reading textbooks is like going to sea without charts, but to study without dealing with patients is not to go to sea at all*
Sir William Osler (1849–1919)
– said to be the most outstanding medical educator of his time

*The secret of patient care is caring for patients*
Peabody

# Post-mortems

The usual advice is probably to avoid these completely, but we all know that in the real world it is difficult to do that. The best thing to do after an exam is to jot down what was asked and to prime your friends in the year below with anything useful you have picked up. Jotting down the topics and questions may be useful in various ways, for example I am told there are agencies who even pay you for this information.

# Principle of precession

According to the 'principle of precession' by Buckminster Fuller, we gain many things on the way, in addition to the actual goal itself. The important thing may not be reaching the goal, but how much we learn as we go along the way. The journey is as important in many ways as the piece of paper you are getting at the end.

*The mirror reflects all objects without being sullied*
*The heart of the wise, like a mirror, should reflect all objects without being sullied by any*
Confucius

Confucius did not probably intend a mirror to be a revision aid, but you can write on it with washable ink or stick on a Post-It™ note – *one* fact per mirror – which you never think about again, but as you look at the mirror each day it will indelibly become etched into your long-term memory (passive learning).

# Problems?

*Nothing lasts forever – not even your troubles!*
Arnold Glasgow

*...the problem is not the problem; the problem is the way people cope. This is what destroys people, not the problem. Then when we learn to cope differently, we deal with the problems differently – and they become different*
Virginia Satir

*...the package deal in being human involves problems, and it means we get to love to laugh to cry to try to get up and fall down and to get up again*
Andrew Matthews

*The way I see it, if you want the rainbow, you got to put up with the rain*
Anonymous

*The mud puddles of life are only there to remind you it's just been raining*
Stan Lee

*Obstacles are things a person sees when he takes his eyes off his goal*
E. Joseph Cossman

*It is no good crying over spilt milk because all the forces of the Universe were bent on spilling it*
William Somerset Maugham

*If opportunity doesn't knock, build a door*
Milton Berle

# Record cards and Post-It™ notes

Post-It™ notes are quite handy for learning complex topics by breaking them down into smaller parts. One advantage is that they can be arranged in different ways over books, notes, walls, bathroom mirrors, doors, and wallpaper, for example.

Don't have more than one or two facts per note. Keep it simple. Avoid visual indigestion. Likewise only have two or three notes per mirror or door (or posters, even). (A whole wall with dozens of sticky notes on is an inefficient and time-consuming re-hashing process, although it may impress your flatmates!). Within reason of course, you can do whatever you like. You can use the same sticky notes later, as bookmarks in different textbooks – which allows you to passively review the diagram or fact even while you are studying a completely different topic! Neat, huh!

Record cards can be used in a similar way.

As time is limited, once you've put the topic or facts on the record cards (or Post-It™ notes) you should avoid duplication (yawn) by making yet more notes on those same facts. Instead, maximize remembering those facts on your cards by any means necessary. You can use your revision aids while walking or waiting for the bus, or in the dentist's waiting room. Their convenience lies in their portability. Remember that one or two clear bold facts, diagrams or mind-maps per card is enough.

# Regular breaks

We know that it is more efficient to study in sessions of 20–40 minutes and take regular breaks (e.g. 10–20 minutes). Yep, we talked about breaks earlier!

As well as keeping up your energy levels, and giving you a chance to share ideas and mnemonics with your friends, breaks allow you to *review* the stuff you just learnt and *overview* the stuff you going to learn. Do this at the beginnings and ends of your study sessions.

Many find they get their best ideas and brain waves when they are most relaxed (e.g. in the shower, loo, bed, etc.). When you relax, you go into an alpha-wave state where you are at your most creative.

*We have the best results in our life when we are prepared to go with the flow. This means finding the delicate and elusive balance between effort and relaxation, between attachment and letting go…Relax and let go – go with the flow*

Andrew Matthews

# Review, review, review!

This is the *single most important* study secret. You will notice that reviewing is the fundamental ingredient of all revision strategies.

So how does one review? Any way you like, although a few useful ways are to spend a few minutes (no more!) doing one of these things:

- Scribble down a mind-map (2 minutes).
- Visually scan over the material in your mind's eye.

- Flick through your Post-it™ notes or record cards.
- You can even go through your textbook or notes again (provided you only look *quickly* at the facts you have highlighted or underlined).

So when should you review? Ideally:

- At the start of your session (do a quick mental 2-minute overview of what you know of the topic – even if you think you don't know anything; it is permissible to look at past papers/previous years' tasks instead).
- After every paragraph or every few key facts (if paragraphs are irrelevant).
- At the end of the session (do a quick 2-minute visual fast-forward in your mind, like scanning on a video).
- After 24 hours.
- After 1 week.
- After 1 month.
- Pre-exam (this is usually the only time anybody else does it!).

Reviewing like this takes effort and seems to slow you down – but all this reviewing doesn't mean you need to spend hours slogging through lots of facts. Once you have gone through the material initially, you only need to review your key words, facts and phrases.

# Reward

*The highest reward for a person's toil is not what they get for it, but what they became by it*

John Ruskin

# Small is beautiful!

- Small *is* beautiful in the world of MBBS revision – get the smallest book on the topic. You always have lots of other information sources available, e.g. tutorials, handouts, friends, Internet, etc.
- Only use the minimal number of books per topic – a standard text, a crammer and a revision Q&A-type book is probably too much (but I will forgive you!).
- Study groups can delegate workload to different students – you then teach each other. This is a terrific way to cover large amounts of material in a short time.

# Smile similes

*Smile – it'll increase your face value*

*Smile and the whole world will smile with you*

*Smile – It'll squeeze out endorphins from those reluctant neurones*

*'Coz you smile when you feel good*
*And you feel good*
*When you smile*

Various contributors

# Staggering sessions

This does not refer to what you do on your way back from the medical school bar!

Staggering sessions means that you alternate your subjects. Study at least two topics at one sitting and make sure these are as dissimilar as possible. So, for instance, study anatomy for an hour or so, then alternate it with sociology and then biochemistry, before going back to anatomy.

You'll keep your mental energy levels up this way, while covering the same volume of material – and you'll retain more. This is because you'll avoid the fatigue associated with boredom. It gives those crucial neurons in the relevant section of your brain an hour's rest before returning back to the original topic – as we know, different memories and different subjects use different section of the brain. It is thus useful to know a variety of study methods.

# Sticky wicket?

*The man who removes a mountain begins by carrying away small stones*
Chinese proverb

*Commonsense is genius dressed in its working clothes*
Emerson

*Success is more attitude than aptitude*
Anonymous

*Failure lies not in falling down but in not getting up*
Traditional Chinese proverb

*Life can only be understood backwards; but it must be lived forwards*
Soren Kierkegaard

*Experience, the name men give to their mistakes*
Oscar Wilde

# Study methods

Use any combination of study methods and keep them flexible!

Studying (like medicine) is really more of an art than a science. There are no absolutes! Be as flexible as you like…as *long as you take regular breaks and frequently review* really any study method will work.

Suggestions include Tony Buzan's 'organic' method. This has defined stages including overview, preview, in-view, review, etc. This means each topic is covered several times, looking at different aspects and different levels of detail each time. Other versions include the SQ3R – **s**urvey, **q**uestion, **r**ead, **r**ecite and **r**evise.

The secret is to find the most appropriate method for you, for that topic, for that time, and for that place – *as long as you take regular breaks and review often*.

# Summarize

It has been said that you know you have learnt a topic if you can condense a huge wodge of notes down to the size of a postage stamp!

In practice, if you can summarize all the material from one subject into a few pages or cards, you can be sure you will have understood the material. Then you only need to memorize the key facts. These key facts can be put onto a mind-map for at-a-glance overview and review.

Effective summarizing explains the popularity of finals revision courses which condense the whole MBBS clinical course into a weekend – with good results.

So summarize. Summarize your summary, then summarize that. Then teach it to your colleagues and let them return the favour on another topic you don't have time for.

# Taking yourself too seriously

It is *only* an exam!

Keep things in perspective. Are you filling your mind with gloomy mental pictures? What a waste! This is a symptom of taking yourself too seriously!

If you want to exaggerate and magnify vivid images in your mind, make sure they are of nice things in the world around you, all the positive things that have happened and will happen. Or of fabulous mnemonics to learn things fast and laid back!

And if you were really convinced you were going to re-sit your exam, well revise anyway, because you will still need to learn the stuff.

But, if you are really desperate to be serious about anything, be serious about humour!

*But it does move*

Galileo

# Texts are tools!

Your texts are your tools and your servants – not the other way around!
It is better to get your own books and **highlight**, underline, make notes in the margin, cross out waffly paragraphs, and whittle the words down to what is useful *now* to *you*.

Doing all this will help you learn because it uses visual, motor and audiological (say it to yourself, make tapes, use music…) memory banks all firing simultaneously.

A lot of the excess words are there to help you understand; many wasted words in those big books are the writer's personal view of the Universe – forget all that! Remember what you need to help you gain useful knowledge in the most useful way to get *marks*…

The text is your slave!

*We get taught a lot of things that are never useful*

Richard Bandler

# Wisdom and knowledge

*One of the greatest pieces of economic wisdom is to know what you do not know*

John Kenneth Galbraith

*Can your learned head take leaven*
*From the wisdom of your heart?*

Lao Tse (translated by Witter Bynner)

And finally…

*They know enough*
*who know how to learn*

Henry Adams

Enjoy!

# INDEX